THE WELL-TUNED
BODY

Banish back pain with gentle exercises
based on the ALEXANDER technique

PENNY INGHAM & COLIN SHELBOURN

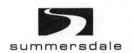

summersdale

THE WELL-TUNED BODY

First published as THE BUSY BODY by Summersdale Publishers Ltd, 2002
This edition copyright © Penny Ingham and Colin Shelbourn 2007

The rights of Penny Ingham and Colin Shelbourn to be identified as the authors of this work have been asserted in accordance with sections 77 and 78 of the Copyright, Designs and Patents Act 1988.

Summersdale Publishers l
46 West Street
Chichester
West Sussex
PO19 1RP
UK

www.summersdale.com

Printed and bound in Great Britain

ISBN: 1-84024-578-6
ISBN 13: 978-1-84024-578-3

THE WELL-TUNED BODY
Penny Ingham and Colin Shelbourn

To Polly and Russell,
for giving me direction (PI)

To Mary, onward and upward (CS)

CONTENTS

INTRODUCTION

How are you holding this book? Is your chin jutting out? Head pulled back? Shoulders hunched? If you are standing, is all the weight on one leg? How are your hips? Hitched to one side? Is your lower back tight?

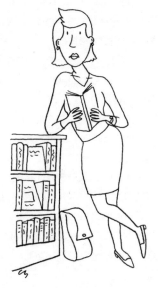

If you are sitting, are you arching your back or slumping in the chair? And by the way, how is your breathing?

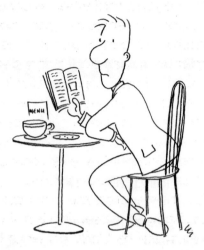

Do you suffer from backache, tiredness, stiffness in the joints, digestive problems, lack of energy, shortness of breath, onset of RSI (Repetitive Strain Injury), irritability, or low self-esteem? If you have answered yes to some or all of these questions, you need *The Well-tuned Body*.

The way that we habitually stand, sit and move can cause all the symptoms above. Few of us have the alert, easy posture we had as children. Over the years we have acquired damaging postural habits which incorporate and reinforce the strain and tension of everyday living. But because we have learnt these habits, we can unlearn them.

Difficult or impossible though this seems, one remarkable man, F. Mathias Alexander, did just that. Alexander (1869–1955) was an Australian actor who developed a persistent vocal problem. Acutely observant, he set out to identify the cause for himself. He noticed that whenever he prepared to speak he became tense. Anyone might observe that in themselves and in others in a general way, but Alexander noticed particular details. Using mirrors, he saw himself pulling back his head, raising his chest and becoming shorter in stature as he prepared to speak. He further observed that, to a greater or lesser degree, this very negative pattern was present in many everyday actions and that most of us carry these patterns of tension in our bodies until they produce pain and impaired movement. Of course, observing is not enough. At first he tried to *make* his body do what he wanted but this only created more tension. Realising this, he set about creating a technique for the re-education of his body, essentially a programme of consciously noticing and inhibiting habitual responses and directing his body to a much more natural and poised way of being. He went on to teach his methods to others and the Alexander technique is now taught worldwide.

HOW TO USE THIS BOOK

This book does not set out to teach the Alexander technique (for that you would need to have lessons with a qualified teacher) but it is based on Alexander's principles. It is important that you should read Chapters 1 to 4 before going on to other sections. These chapters form the foundation of the book and are fundamental to understanding later chapters. Begin with these and then you are ready to dip into any of the remaining chapters in or out of sequence, with the exception of Chapter 16, which should be read when you have looked at the book as a whole. Each chapter can be used as a self-contained piece of work but your understanding will build up chapter by chapter.

Appendix 1 – Body Map – is also essential if you want to successfully navigate round your body.

Each chapter contains five sections: The Problem, The Exercises, The Principle, The Posture Post-it and Reorganise Your Life.

 ## THE PROBLEM

An unwelcome symptom such as backache is your body giving you useful feedback. Listen to it. The aches, pains and stiffness may well be the result of something you are doing to yourself. Over the years, you may have acquired damaging postural habits or methods of working and moving which put unnecessary strain on your body. But, if you are doing harm to yourself, you can learn to undo it. What you need is this book and a little insight, patience and perseverance.

It is important to realise that body problems are interrelated. That stiffness in your fingers, for example, may be caused by the way you sit. The symptoms listed in this section are a rough indicator of what might be going wrong; all the chapters in the book will be beneficial, even if you think you need to address only one particular problem.

 THE EXERCISES

These are quite unlike conventional keep-fit exercises. They are habit-breakers. They require mental rather than physical effort. They are designed to examine and remedy the tense and over-effortful way in which you have been making everyday actions, and to encourage your body to revert to its natural, tension-free way of doing things. Take your time over each exercise – if you do it too quickly, your muscles will take over and repeat the old, habitual way of doing things.

Throughout this book, we use words and images which help you make less effort. For example we say: 'Let your elbows drop to your sides', 'Allow your shoulders to widen', 'Think of a string taking the crown of your head upwards'. All these phrases help you to naturally adopt these ideas, which is the very opposite of forcing the body into a good posture.

When you attempt the exercises, do so with a positive and interested attitude. The quality of your attention is a key factor in the effectiveness of each exercise. If you perform them quickly in a let's-get-this-done sort of way, your body will miss the point. Staying with the process can be difficult at first. If you find that your mind is elsewhere, find another time when you are in a more receptive mood. Work on these exercises when you feel you can give them your full attention and then you will be making real changes.

Remember that just as you acquired damaging postural habits by repeating the same thing over and over again, so you need to unlearn the habits by repeating the exercises. Like skilled craftsmen or musicians you never stop practising. Continue to work on yourself.

 ## THE PRINCIPLE

In this section we explain more about why and how you might have acquired a particular problem and the relevance of the exercises. It puts the work you are doing into a useful context. You will find it helpful to read these sections along with a glance at the Body Map.

 ## THE POSTURE POST-IT

The chapter in a nutshell – thoughts you repeat to yourself to direct your body into its easier, natural posture. They act as antidotes to bad postural habits and reinforce the new you.

They work in a similar way to affirmations. They help to change the unhelpful script most of us have running around our heads most of the time (for example substituting the positive 'I can do this' for the negative 'I can't do that'). Repetition is the key factor to affirmations; the positive thought consciously replaces the negative until a new way of thinking is formed.

Thoughts work on our body in a similar, very potent way. The Post-its help remind you of useful thoughts on posture. We offer some suggestions for these but feel free to add your own – making up your own will help you think about the work you are doing on yourself. But keep them positive – 'do' is more useful than 'don't' and is less likely to introduce the wrong idea. For instance, if we say: 'Don't think of an elephant!' what is the first thing you think of? Exactly.

Once you have your thoughts, distribute them about your desk, computer screen, your fridge door; anywhere you will see and be reminded of them.

REORGANISE YOUR LIFE

In this section there are practical tips and hints on how to modify your lifestyle and environment to help maintain the new you. Be a rugged individualist; look after yourself in a practical, organised way and get back in control of your body.

... AND FINALLY

Once you understand the problems poor body use can cause, you can use that understanding to get back in control of your busy life. Furthermore, the principles in *The Well-tuned Body* can be incorporated into your everyday actions. Whatever you are doing, you can be using the ideas in this book to make yourself feel better, fresher, more in control and more energetic. *The Well-tuned Body* sets out a programme for change. It is a body owner's handbook to help you regain and maintain ease, poise and pain-free movement. Although you can treat the exercises individually, their effect is cumulative. Any of the exercises will be a useful re-education of your body, performed wherever, whenever you can. The more you practise, the more you get out of it. It's not just about work or play – it's about life.

CHAPTER 1

ANYONE FOR TENSION?

THE PROBLEM

Are you doing too much?

Most of us are tense to a degree – you might be breathless, have a bad back, headache, digestion problems or just feel more tired than you think you should be. You're doing too much.

It's nothing to do with a heartless boss or unsympathetic co-workers, it's you! You can be lying on the beach and still be doing too much. It's all down to the habits you've learned since you were a child.

THE EXERCISES

Exercise 1:

To begin with, here's a really easy demonstration of muscle tension and how to release it. (This is also a good exercise in observation.)

Hold your hand (either one will do) in front of you at face level, palm side-on, forearm vertical. Your wrist needs to be visible for this exercise.

Keeping your hand open, tighten your wrist muscles. You will feel a pull towards your elbow. Notice that this measurably shortens the distance between the tips of your fingers and your elbow, and arches your hand.

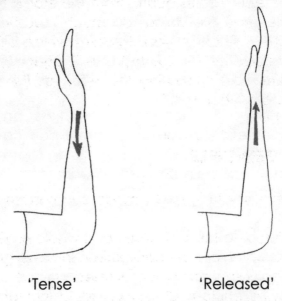

'Tense'   'Released'

Now release the muscle tension. Your hand is still supported in an upright position, but you are doing much less work and the distance between your fingertips and elbow is much longer. You've released tension to allow your hand and forearm to lengthen upwards.

This is a precise analogy of everything postural we will learn during the course of this book.

Exercise 2:
Sit at a table with a cup in front of you. Keeping your elbows clear of the table, place your left hand on your right bicep and pick up the cup with your right hand. (If you are left-handed, reverse this.) Bring the cup to your lips. How much effort do you need?

If you feel muscles pulling from the elbow to the shoulder, you are doing too much. You have a nice little muscle in your forearm which is more than adequate for the task. Try it again on the opposite side, minimising the effort all the time. Hinge, don't heave.

 PRINCIPLE

Tension – what is it and why do our muscles grow tense?

We become tense at work for a whole variety of reasons which can be categorised into two groups – psychological and physical (mechanical).

Some psychological factors would include: not

enough personal space on the tube, not enough office space, the urge to leave the meeting NOW and not being able to, the primitive urge to have a punch-up with someone at the meeting when politeness and promotion prospects prohibit us.

Physical factors would include: chairs sloping the wrong way (see Chapter 5), unsatisfactory work stations, cramped working conditions and so on.

When tense, the posture we adopt is the startle response. That is, whatever the stimulus, we respond in the same way: we tighten our necks, pull our heads back and shorten the whole length of our spines. We have entered 'flight or fight' mode. We make these unnecessary and damaging movements whenever we make an action – however minor. We've learnt the habit – through repetition in formative years – of gearing ourselves up, ready for action, instead of going smoothly into that action.

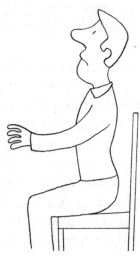

When we're psychologically tense, our muscles are tense. One way to help cope with the psychological pressure is to begin to deal with the muscular tension. For example, unclench that jaw. If your jaw is tight, the rest of your body cannot be relaxed – other muscles will tighten as well; it is a cumulative effect.

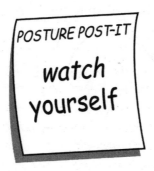

 REORGANISE YOUR LIFE

Give yourself time to observe these energy-wasting habits. Do a personal tension audit: when you make a move, perform an action or respond to a request, stop, relax, observe what you're about to do and break the habit of tension.

When you're busy at work, it is easy to forget about your body unless it becomes stiff or painful. But you don't have to ignore your body in order to concentrate on something else. To begin with, you may need to take time out to observe what you

23

are doing. As you become more practised, you will be more aware of how you are moving, sitting or standing whilst engaged in everyday activities. It is a skill which can be learned – a slightly different mode of thinking with continuing benefits.

CHAPTER 2

FIRST STOP
AND THINK

THE PROBLEM

You want to stop being tense but you don't know how. People tell you to relax but no matter how you try, somehow it eludes you. So how do you do it? This chapter gives you the first step.

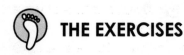 **THE EXERCISES**

Exercise 1:

You can do this sitting or standing. Cross your arms. Now cross them the other way. Not so easy is it? Notice how much you had to reorganise your approach and think through the movement before crossing your arms in the unaccustomed way.

Make a point of trying a few actions with your non-dominant side, for example: which arm goes into the jacket first? Same hand on the computer mouse? Telephone always on the same side? Trousers on with the same leg first? You have to think it through to reorganise these activities to favour your non-dominant side. This will make you more sensitive to body balance.

Exercise 2:

For this you need a small, unbreakable object such as a ball of paper or a plastic cup. Standing or sitting, prepare to throw the object from one hand to the other. Extend the catching hand out in front of you. Usually you would move this hand to catch the object but in this exercise you choose not to – you let it remain still.

With your throwing hand, throw the object into your catching hand without moving the latter. The object may fall but never mind. If it lands in your hand, clasp it, but if it misses, let it go. Under no circumstances are you to move your catching hand to intercept the object. The purpose of this exercise is to test your ability to resist the impulse to move.

Try this a few times with both your dominant and non-dominant hand doing the throwing. As with the previous exercise you will find you have to engage your brain to actively inhibit the catching reflex.

 ## THE PRINCIPLE

Stopping and thinking are twin activities which should be complementary.

Stopping – putting a pause in between resolving to make an action and then performing it – allows for thinking time. You can then act in the newly organised, unfamiliar way. In exercise 1 you have to *think* how , for example, to fold your arms the opposite way and in exercise 2 you have to consciously inhibit your usual catching movement and change to a new use of your catching hand. Difficult, yes, but *not* impossible!

As you work your way through this book, you will find that you are being encouraged to pause (inhibit your reflexes), think about what you are about to do and direct your body to go about the action in the new way (sometimes using images as a tool to help you).

In this way, you will find that you do not have to be a slave to damaging postural habits. You can learn to observe, think about what you are doing and reorganise the way you are about to do it.

By making your mind work harder, your body will have an easier time.

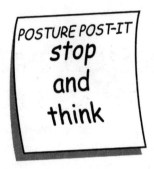

 REORGANISE YOUR LIFE

Begin by organising the filing cabinet inside your head. Dispose of outdated notions of posture. Posture which requires strenuous effort (chin up, chest out) can go straight in the bin. Instead, start working with the idea that to achieve poise, balance and elegance of movement, you can do less work by thinking in a new way about your body. The exercises, thoughtfully performed, will help you recognise when you are making too much effort.

Thinking organises your body to do less, not more.

CHAPTER 3

IS WORK A PAIN IN THE NECK?

THE PROBLEM

Do you suffer from a stiff neck or tension headaches – for example, when sitting at a desk or keyboard?

You're probably tensing your neck and pulling your head back, without realising it. If your neck is tight, your chin juts forward and you're compressing your spine. You're probably so used to this posture that it feels completely normal. Sitting up straight is the usual reaction but this is not a good way to go about it and is more effort; you need to attend to the way you balance your head on your neck.

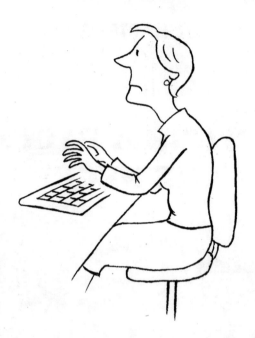

 THE EXERCISES

Exercise 1:

Begin by sitting on an office chair or dining chair (not your favourite armchair). Imagine a string attached to the crown of your head and going up to the ceiling. (The crown is not the top of your head – it is farther back.)

A friendly puppeteer is about to pull on the string, to draw you gently upwards, crown first. As the puppeteer pulls, your neck begins to lengthen. This will make you aware of the muscles at the back of your neck. Think of these muscles relaxing.

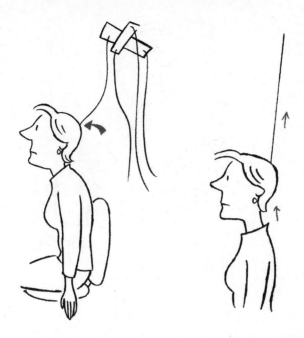

As the neck muscles release and lengthen, the back of your neck can't help but move towards the back of your collar and as your crown is drawn upwards, your chin drops and your forehead rolls slightly forward.

By imagining a puppeteer doing the work, you are not stiffening or forcing your neck into a new position but allowing it to happen naturally. The less you tighten the back of your neck, the longer it becomes; muscles contract as you tighten them and lengthen when they relax.

As your neck muscles relax and lengthen, your head, neck and back realign themselves and you regain your natural poise.

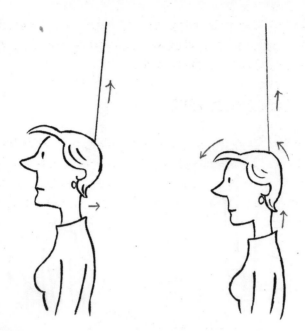

Exercise 2:

Find a hand mirror and a larger mirror. Turn your back on the large mirror and align the hand mirror to view the reflection of the back of your neck in the large mirror.

Now think through the images in Exercise 1.

Notice that if you don't stiffen your neck but allow it to release upwards, it will ease back into your collar, your head will roll very slightly forward (as if rather more weight has dropped into your forehead) and, as your neck muscles continue to release tension, you will see that you have rather more back of neck. You will find that the more you think of releasing those neck muscles, rather than tightening them in a 'sit up straight' manner, the longer your neck and spine become. This is a very useful look and learn exercise.

 THE PRINCIPLE

Your head weighs around five kilograms. We're so used to this weight that we don't notice it. Next time you're in the supermarket, pick up five kilogram bags of sugar; that's what your neck has to carry every day.

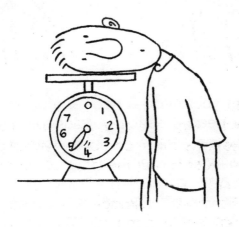

Your head is carried on the top of your spine. It balances at the atlanto-occipital joint, the uppermost joint of your spine, deep inside your head. This joint is perhaps higher in the skull than you imagined.

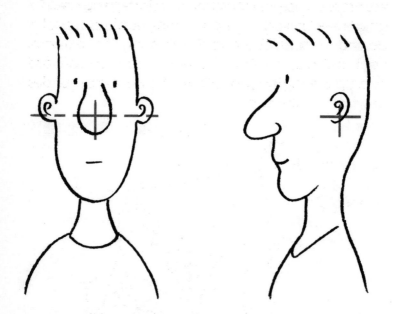

The front of your head is heavier than the back. When your head is perfectly balanced, this extra weight rolls your forehead slightly forward at the pivot, the atlanto-occipital joint.

In everyday life, most of us tend to carry our heads poorly balanced: chin forward, neck compressed, taking the world on the chin. To see what is wrong with this we need to add that there are two layers of muscles involved in the head, neck and back. One layer is the external musculature, the other is the internal, postural musculature. We don't need to tighten the external muscles to balance our heads when we're in our normal, upright position (sitting or standing). If we do tighten these external muscles, we are making unnecessary and damaging stressful effort. We should let the internal postural muscles do the work. In Exercise 2, releasing the external neck muscles so that the head can roll forward and up is exactly what allows the postural muscles to work unimpeded.

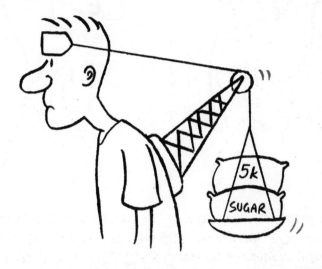

When our muscles release, they lengthen. If your neck muscles are released, you cannot help but be taller. By allowing the crown of your head to release up, your head rolls slightly forward and your neck – which was tightened – begins to ease back and straighten. With the pressure off, your neck and the full extent of your spine lengthen and realign. Balancing your head becomes effortless. You are more relaxed, taller, you look leaner and you are feeling better already.

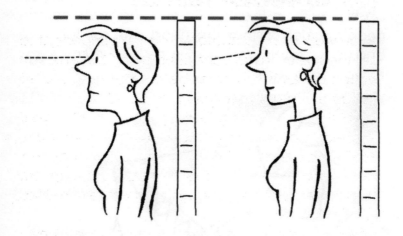

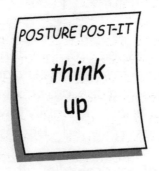

REORGANISE YOUR LIFE

If you work at a computer screen, it's important to get the screen in the correct position. This has been written about many times before but now you've got a new factor to take into account.

Once you've lengthened your neck, your forehead has rolled slightly forwards and your eye level is no longer where it was. In fact, it may feel very unfamiliar – as though you are peering out from under your eyelashes. Expect this to take time to become familiar.

If your screen was previously correctly positioned (and that's a big if) you'll now find it needs to be lowered.

Before you start heaving the screen about, try it with a book. Open the book, then hold it at arm's length where your screen is now. Focus on a word or phrase, then lower the book as you lengthen your neck. Feel where the book is most comfortable to read. That's where your screen should be.

By the way, this does not mean that you must hold your head vertical at all times. You can move your head to look around you, but make sure it always comes back to the vertical resting place. With released neck muscles and a balanced head, it is easy to move your head naturally when required. (Practise now for Chapter 8!)

CHAPTER 4

RECHARGING THE BATTERIES

THE PROBLEM

Fatigued, lack of stamina, bone tired, the Monday morning feeling which lasts all week?

You probably won't realise it unless your back is giving you pain, but those feelings of fatigue are most likely coming from your spine.

Apart from sleeping at night, how many times do you lie down in any 24 hour period? What everyone's spine needs is a 20 minute period of lying down, ideally twice during the working day – once around lunch time and again five hours later.

THE EXERCISE

You will need a clear floor space which is warm and comfortable to lie on. You also need a small stack of paperback books or magazines to support your head and, ideally, 20 minutes (although even five minutes is beneficial). Not all workplaces have a clear floor space but you can usually find somewhere (a meeting room, the chairman's office). Don't be self-conscious – it is important to do this around the middle of the day.

Lie down on your back, with your head resting on the stack of books and your knees pointing towards the ceiling.

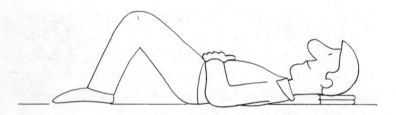

Your head should be supported by the books with your neck clear of the floor. The contact point with the books is the lower, flatter part of the back of your head, just below the bump of the occiput. (The bony protuberance at the back of the head – see Appendix 1.)

Adjust the height of the stack to establish head, neck and back alignment; with too few books, your chin will stick up towards the ceiling, with too many your chin will press down into your throat. The books should support your head in such a way that your chin tilts slightly towards your chest with a gentle slope from forehead to chin.

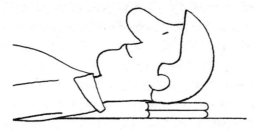

A good rule of thumb is that the back of your neck is approximately parallel to the floor; you can check this by running three or four fingers between your neck and the floor, making a note of the height of the stack for next time.

Let your elbows rest on the floor as far out to the side as possible, with your hands resting palms down on your body, just below the rib cage. Relax your wrists and feel the full weight of your hands on your body – take your time over this and feel the tension dropping out of your wrists.

Place your feet on the floor as near to your bottom as feels comfortable, without strain, with the inside of your feet in line with the outside of your hips.

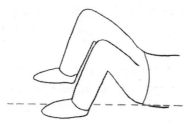

Your knees point to the ceiling. Relax your leg muscles so your kneecaps are over your little toes; if you are too tense, your knees will pull together and the kneecaps will be over your big toes. This is quite a subtle point but a good indicator of how relaxed your leg muscles have become. As with the wrists, spend time working on this.

When your knees are at a point of balance, you may feel them trembling slightly. This is usual – as you practise, you'll achieve the right point without the trembling. You are learning quite a sophisticated balancing act.

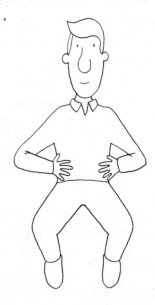

Relax your ankles and bring your attention to the underside of your feet; if your legs are appropriately balanced, the weight will distribute around the outside of your feet – a perfect footprint – and not down on the arch. Now you can begin!

To bring yourself into the present moment and closer to your sensations – listen.

Absorb the sounds around you as though you are collecting them. Some will be sounds from the room around you, some from outside and some will be the sounds of your own body, such as your breathing.

Now think of your spine releasing tension and your body lengthening and widening. Feel the support of the floor beneath you and think of sinking into soft sand, your body imprint getting longer and wider. As you lose tension, you make more contact with the surface beneath you.

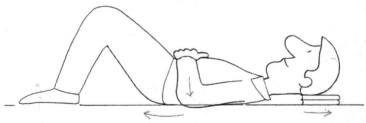

If you are finding all of this difficult to visualise, you might find the following suggestion useful. Ask yourself, now that you are lying down, how you know that the surface you are lying on is a carpet or a rug? Of course, you would have been able to see what it was before you lay down, but now, how do you know that the books supporting your head are hard and the rug is soft? What tells you that the texture of one is different from the other? What is the temperature beneath your feet compared to that under your body and under your head? All of these questions will help you get in touch with your sensations by focusing your thoughts on what you can feel now, in this moment.

Lying in semi-supine, these thoughts can be extended into other useful thought exercises to enhance the very useful work that is already benefiting your back. Try picturing a line connecting two joints of your body; for example, your right knee and left shoulder. Imagine that line becoming longer as your muscles release.

Now switch your attention to your right wrist and left shoulder. Again, picture the line connecting them becoming longer.

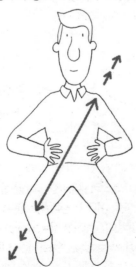

Work around your whole body in this manner, not forgetting the many joints in your feet and hands and the 24 joints of your spine, extending up into your skull. It does not matter too much which joints you choose – they can be next to each other or on opposite sides of the body – the benefit is the same.

As you can see, if any colleagues ask what you are doing, you are perfectly justified in telling them: 'working!'

THE PRINCIPLE

The discs of your spine perform the vital function of insulating your vertebrae from physical trauma (the everyday impact of moving around). The discs are like sponges, absorbing spinal fluid to act as highly efficient shock absorbers.

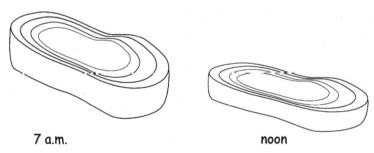

7 a.m.   noon

After five hours of being upright, they need recharging to maintain their resilience. Without this recharging, after a further five hours the discs will have compressed even further, lost fluid and be well below optimum condition. They will now be much less resilient than when you got out of bed in the morning. This is one reason why most people lose measurable height during the course of a day.

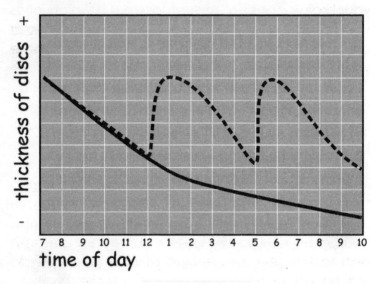

without lying down ━━━━━━━━

result of lying in semi-supine -------

During a typical working day, what do we do? Most of us spend hours at a desk, sitting in meetings or in a vehicle or otherwise remaining upright. So long as we stay vertical, the essential process of disc recharging cannot happen.

Lie down in the semi-supine position described above and three things happen:

At a mechanical level, the discs absorb the fluid they need and are once more able to perform their important task – along with the vertebrae – of forming a protective tunnel for the spinal cord, from which nerves run linking every part of your body to your brain.

Secondly, by lying in the semi-supine position and using the floor as a reference, you can feel where your back is over-arched (as in Fig. A).

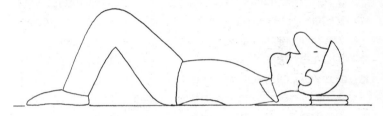

Fig. A

Your spine is naturally gently curved for strength and resilience – so gently that your back should feel flat on the floor when your knees are raised.

The more the underside of your body contacts the floor, the less tense you are. Tension would have you arching away from the floor. The books help you realign your head, neck and back.

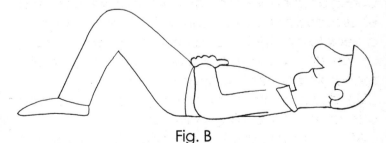

Fig. B

Turn this book through 90 degrees to show the lying figure (Fig. B) upright, and you will see how your back should look whilst you are sitting (see Chapter 5).

Finally, when you get up again, having realigned your head, neck and back, lengthened and widened your body and having recharged the discs of your spine, you will be feeling much clearer, more relaxed and focused. And, incidentally, you will be taller! The combination of plumped up discs and muscle lengthening can restore your height by as much as three centimetres. Your discs recharge as you work on releasing tension from your muscles. You are effectively working and relaxing at the same time.

As you learn to release muscle tension, you will remain taller during the course of the day and so have less height to regain during the lying down work. The mechanical advantages of lying down are still vital to the well-being of your spine and so to the well-being of you. Remember that your discs still need regular rehydrating.

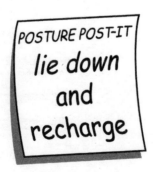

POSTURE POST-IT
*lie down
and
recharge*

REORGANISE YOUR LIFE

Finding both the time and a place to lie down may be difficult. At home, the place is not likely to be a problem; and at work you can usually find somewhere to lie down. As for time, rather than have a coffee break, have a lying down break – the benefits will be far greater.

Having understood the principles and experienced the effects, you will feel confident enough to make this lying down work an essential part of your life. Make a point of putting it in your diary or organiser. You will be valuing yourself, improving your personal performance and your colleagues will respond positively to that.

You will also gain benefits if you can schedule a brief session of lying down work before tackling something stressful or demanding – for example, before an important meeting – especially if it has been a long time since your last session. You will feel clearer and more capable before tackling the challenge.

Make sure your work schedule allows for time to work on yourself.

CHAPTER 5

ARE YOU SITTING COMFORTABLY?

THE PROBLEM

Most of us sit badly. Problems associated with poor sitting include fatigue, lower back problems, sciatic pain, poor breathing, bad digestion, poor circulation and lumber disc problems.

 All these problems can be caused by faulty posture whilst sitting. Sitting puts three times the strain on your spine as standing (and we shouldn't stand for long, either... but see Chapter 10 for more about that).

THE EXERCISES

Exercise 1:

Most of us don't know how to sit and it takes practice. You might find that sitting in a poised, balanced and less stressful way seems so unfamiliar – and uses your back muscles in such a different way – that it feels uncomfortable at first.

Find a chair with as firm a seat as possible – note that it's what you sit on that's important, not the chair back. The seat should be horizontal or, ideally, slightly sloping downwards from back to front (never the other way round).

When sitting, your legs should be at right angles to your body or, ideally, your hips higher than your knees. Your feet should be comfortably apart, fully supported by the floor.

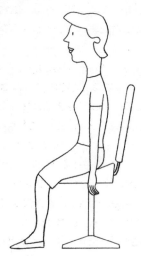

ARE YOU SITTING COMFORTABLY?

Sitting on the chair, first find your sit bones by turning your hands palms up and sitting on them. Feel the sharper sit bones towards the back of the base of your bottom.

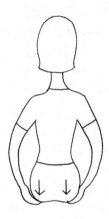

Now you remove your hands. Let the weight of your torso be fully and equally supported down through your sit bones – think of them as little feet in your bottom.

Slide a hand down the length of your spine until the palm rests on the sacrum and your middle finger on the coccyx, or tailbone. (See Appendix 1 – Body Map.) Allow the whole of this area to drop by releasing the muscles. Your buttocks will release outwards, like an inverted fan opening. You will begin to feel your sit bones contacting the chair more fully. This will seem unfamiliar if you associate good sitting with the classroom technique of tightening muscles to sit bolt upright.

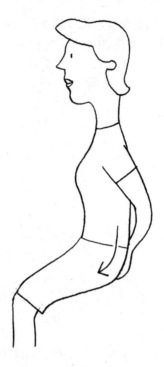

You can actually feel the tension dropping out of your back as your tailbone drops. If your back feels slumped, it is because you are forgetting to allow your neck to lengthen and your head to roll forward and upwards. The release of muscle tension and alignment of your head, neck and back are crucial and indispensable parts of sitting comfortably.

Think of both your neck and tailbone lengthening out of your spine.

Although you may associate the relaxing of your lower back with slumping, the important difference is in the buoyancy of your head as it balances on the top of your lengthening spine.

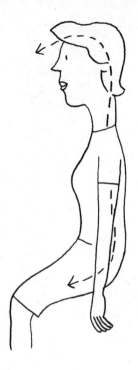

Exercise 2:

Put one hand on the front of your body, just under your breastbone. Allow yourself to push your chin forward and pull your head back to go into the old, bad way of sitting. Feel how this pushes that area of your gut down. Is it any wonder we get stomach problems through bad posture?

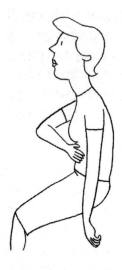

Now try this: put both hands on your sides, spanning the distance between the bottom of your ribs and the top of your pelvis.

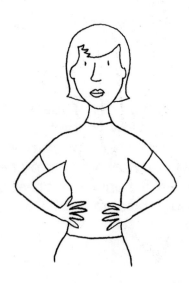

The more space there is there, the better. And if you find one side has less space than the other, then this reflects an asymmetrical sitting position. To correct this, think of your head and spine as a plumb line passing down through your body and that you are sitting equally on both sit bones.

Exercise 3:

Now redirect your attention to your legs and feet. When you're sitting, your other important area of support is the floor. If your legs are balanced and supported, your knees will slightly drift out from the centre line. Think of your knees in relation to your toes. In good sitting, your kneecaps should be over your little toes, not over your big toes.

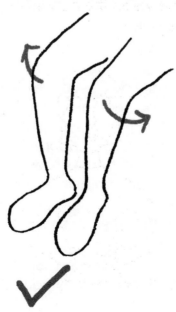

Try tightening your legs together – as though clutching a champagne bottle between your knees – then release them and you'll notice that your knees naturally drift away from each other.

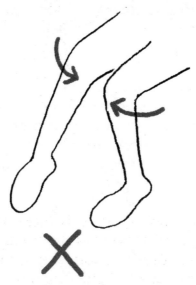

You may find that you need to relax your ankles to let the soles of your feet remain in full contact with the floor.

Now with your torso supported by the chair, your feet supported by the floor and your head balanced, you really are sitting comfortably.

 THE PRINCIPLE

Sitting is a whole body thing. Your head and pelvis balance each other and they can do it wrongly:

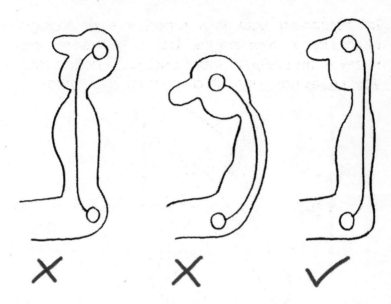

Even in poised sitting there is three times more strain on your spine than when standing. All around your joints there are feedback mechanisms which cause your muscles to tighten when you are off-balance. If you stop fighting gravity and regain your balance, you will be using them less and making much less effort.

Your sit bones, formed from the lower part of your pelvis, are two rockers which make it possible to balance the weight of your torso in sitting. Sitting balanced, the weight of your head is distributed along the whole length of your spine. When we sit badly, that weight falls directly onto the lumber region.

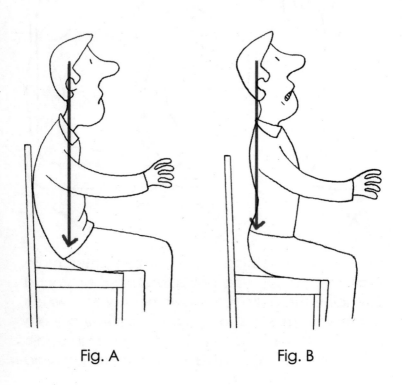

Fig. A   Fig. B

This is a major cause of slipped disc conditions and why they nearly always happen in this part of the spine. You do just as much harm sitting in a self-consciously tense, upright position (as in Fig. B) as you do sitting in a slumped collapse (as in Fig. A).

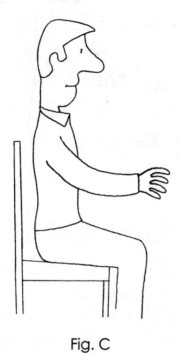

Fig. C

This position (Fig. C) is neither slumped nor strained – it's poised.

Once you get used to the feel of being balanced when you sit, you'll stay relaxed, comfortable and happier for longer.

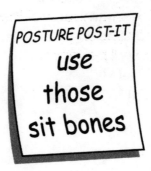

POSTURE POST-IT
use
those
sit bones

 REORGANISE YOUR LIFE

Make sure your chair height is correct – your lower legs should be vertical and your thighs either horizontal or sloping slightly downwards from hips to knees and your feet fully supported by the floor.

If your chair is badly designed, modify it! Invest in a specialist wedge-shaped cushion (or have one made from a block of hard foam) to raise your hips slightly higher than your knees. You may also need to modify the height of your desk.

If your chair's upholstery is very soft – or if your chair seat slopes back – sit on the front edge to support your sit bones. (If your chair is on castors, be very careful how you do this – invest in some carpet protectors to stop your chair sliding backwards.)

Make the surface of your chair support you – if

it is too soft, make a hard cushion from a piece of plywood covered in soft fabric.

It is important to remember that the floor and your chair are there to support you. If you don't accept their support, you will be tense.

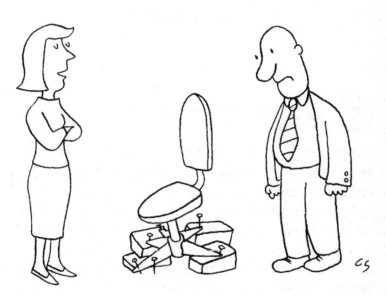

'It might not be very elegant but think how much better I'll look when I'm sitting on it.'

CHAPTER 6

IN THE CHAIR

THE PROBLEM

In the previous chapter, we looked at postural problems whilst sitting in a chair. Those problems (principally of the lower back) are exacerbated when you become active: leaning forward to type, write, read or when getting up and sitting down. The effect is cumulative.

Building on the work in the last chapter, now is the time to take it further and become master of the chair!

THE EXERCISES

Exercise 1:

You can either do this sitting at a desk or table, or by imagining that there is one in front of you. This exercise should take you at least five minutes – do not rush it.

We are going to practise the movement you have to make to go forward from sitting position to, for example, eat, write or work at a desk. For simplicity, leave your hands resting palms up on your lap – at the moment your head, spine and lower body are enough to be thinking about.

Sit on a chair with as firm a seat as possible. Your legs should be at right angles to your body – or, ideally, hips higher than knees – sit bones in contact with the seat of the chair, feet flat on the floor, knees and ankles relaxed, head nicely poised on top of your spine.

Locate your hips. This is important – they are almost certainly not where you think they are. These are not the part of you that holds your trousers up – that's the brim of your pelvis. Your hips are much further down, the bony protuberances at the very top of your legs on the outside, and deep in the groin on the inside.

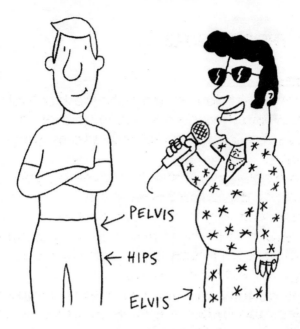

Your hips are the hinges which allow your seated body to go forward to the desk or table. You will be pivoting slowly at your hips; your torso and spine working as one unit.

Now you're ready to begin moving. Work on this exercise very slowly, pausing to organise yourself. The aim is to remain relaxed, aligned, lengthened and poised throughout.

Think of your forehead being magnetised towards the work area of your desk in front of you. You are being drawn forward but with your head, neck and back moving as one. This image will start the momentum and allow your torso to drift gently forwards.

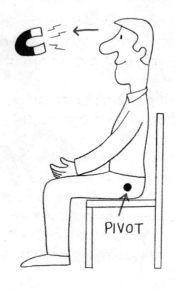

PIVOT

As you go forwards, free your neck and back of tension. We want to maintain the length and freedom we achieved in Chapter 3.

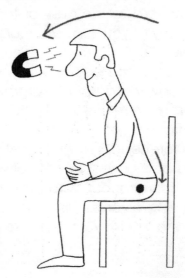

Think of your neck continuing to lengthen and your lower spine – your tailbone – continuing to drop, until you arrive at a position for comfortable working.

Your relaxed legs continue to do nothing, except remain balanced. If your legs tighten, loosen those knees.

The return journey reverses this process; think of the magnet, now behind your head, drawing you back and up as your weight drops slightly more into your tailbone. The counterbalancing effect causes you to rock gently back into the upright sitting position, once more pivoting at your hips.

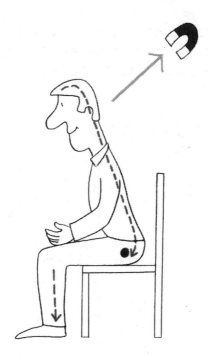

The movement does NOT start by pulling your head back and your chin up, otherwise you will scrunch the back of your neck and arch the small of your back.

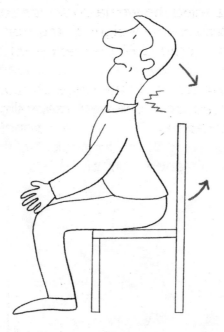

NB: Throughout both parts of the exercise, be careful to notice and avoid the very common tendency to swerve your torso, head or knees to the right or left.

This exercise retrains your body to move much more easily and naturally and without twisting.

Exercise 2:
Standing up from sitting couldn't be simpler but, of course, it could be simpler than we make it.

Sit on the chair as before. Be particularly conscious of the balance of your head on your neck, the chair supporting your torso and the floor under your feet. Think of the undersides of your feet. Although you will be using the whole underside (except the arches) to bear your weight as you stand, most of the weight – around 60 per cent – will be in your heels.

Now move nearer to the edge of your seat and bring your feet back until your heels fall in a line just behind your knees.

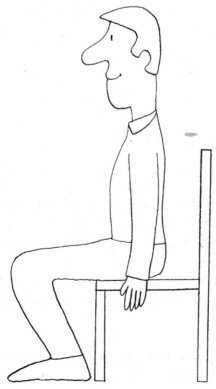

Think through the activity ahead. From sitting to standing requires that you remain balanced all the time and that you go through the process of standing up by leaving one supporting object (the chair) in favour of giving all your weight to the other (the floor).

Think of your forehead being magnetised forwards. Rocking on your sit bones, allow your torso to drift gently forwards until it is sufficiently over your heels for you to straighten your legs easily into the standing position.

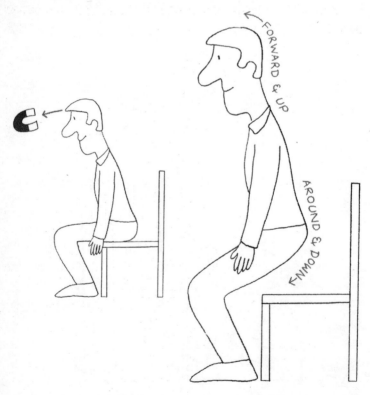

You'll know by now that a common mistake is to start the movement by tightening your neck, pulling back the head and thrusting the chin forward, as though coming up for air. Check that this isn't happening as it can be extraordinarily difficult to resist. Without this tension, you feel light and buoyant as your head leads you forward and upwards.

Keep dropping your tailbone as you stand, with your weight predominantly in your heels.

Sitting down into the chair reverses the process! Think of it as a kind of interrupted squat – the chair being the interruption.

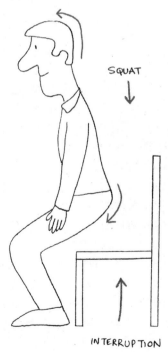

SQUAT

INTERRUPTION

As soon as your bottom reaches the chair seat, let yourself be fully supported again by the chair and the floor. Now you are sitting comfortably again.

Exercise 3:
Try standing up with your eyes shut. You will be much more aware of keeping your balance as you move, a key factor in good posture.

Take note of how you moved. Using these observations, try standing again with your eyes open, incorporating the more secure, and therefore balanced way you moved when you had your eyes shut.

 THE PRINCIPLE

Sitting is not passive. Most of us have developed a range of bad habits associated with sitting, or getting in and out of a chair. The primary bad habit is beginning an action by pulling the head back and tightening the neck.

Having established a balanced sitting posture (as in Chapter 5), learning to move forward in a comfortable, balanced manner provides a foundation for a whole range of further activities.

Unless we're conscious of the way in which we do this, leaning forward falls into the classic stimulus-response pattern; our work is there in front of us and we react by reaching towards it without thinking about how we are getting there. Result – we are using far more effort than we need to for something which is a simple, repetitive and everyday part of our lives.

With the sit bones fully supported by the chair, and your feet supported by the floor, we are perfectly balanced. We don't need to spring into action by getting chin, legs, arms and shoulders involved, simply to lean forward.

Sitting is as much to do with the head as the bottom – remember that the head weighs around five kilograms. Leaning forward is a matter of adjusting your weight slightly and letting gravity do the work. Throughout, we allow the spine to work as one unit, carrying the head and body forward without undue effort.

When we get into a chair in a thoughtless and disorganised way, using our back for support instead of our legs, we stay like that and so retain bad posture.

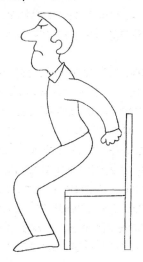
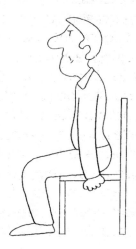

When we get out of the chair in an unbalanced and disorganised way, we are using our spines when we should be using our legs to carry our weight up into standing position.

The job of standing up and sitting down should be done by the legs, not the spine, which should remain at ease throughout.

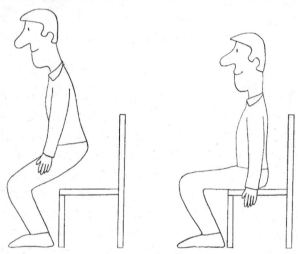

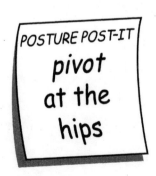

REORGANISE YOUR LIFE

There are some circumstances under which you can reorganise your environment to help you feel more secure when standing up and sitting down: feeling physically secure is a prerequisite for good body use. So, for example, if you have an office chair with castors, restrict them so that the chair does not move when you go to sit down or stand up.

Most importantly of all, don't sit for too long: visit the water cooler more often. If you work at a computer, most machines have an alarm which can be set to chime gently every half hour, reminding you to get up and move around. The more you move, the better. Not only are you avoiding getting fixed in a sitting position, you are giving yourself an opportunity to put into practice the ideas in this book. (for more thoughts about how to incorporate all these ideas into everyday activity, see Chapter 16)

CHAPTER 7

REACH FOR THE PHONE

THE PROBLEM

Middle and lower backache? Pain and stiffness in arms and shoulders?

When we reach and stretch from a sitting position, we can inadvertently put a tremendous strain on our middle and lower back, particularly if the movement is repeated during the course of the day. This, of course, is common when we are sitting at a desk, reaching for the phone, that urgent memo or the coffee cup on the far side of the keyboard.

This is a classic example of how a simple action can cause damage because we do it repeatedly, without thought.

THE EXERCISE

This may seem a very simple, everyday thing to do, but follow the exercise slowly and gently and you will see an immediate benefit.

From a sitting position, you are going to be reaching for an imaginary object just out of reach on your right. Your body will continue to face forwards.

Find a suitable office chair so you can sit and feel the contact of the seat with your sit bones. Your feet should be flat on the floor, the chair and floor fully supporting you (as in Chapter 5).

Drop your hands down by your sides, relax your arms and shoulders, and once again imagine a string taking your head and neck upwards so that your spine lengthens.

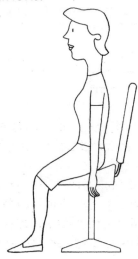

Letting your eyes lead, gently turn your head to the right to look for the object you want to pick up.

Extend your right arm towards the object, an imaginary string leading your fingers towards it. Your shoulder remains relaxed and down – the more your muscles release and your shoulder drops, the longer your reach becomes. Most people simply do not believe this until they have tried it.

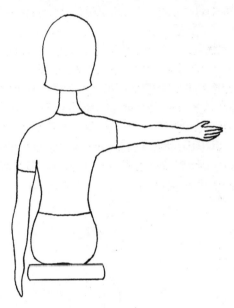

Once you feel that your arm has extended to its fullest amount, then, and only then, begin to gently lean into the movement.

Now, check where those sit bones are. They should both still be in contact with the chair. The likelihood is that the area around your left sit bone has begun to tighten and rise (as in Fig.A).

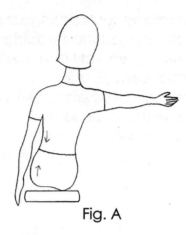

Fig. A

Think of relaxing and dropping this area as you gently lean towards your object.

Keep both sit bones in contact with the chair and you will feel the sides of your torso relaxing. Your reach increases. You are increasing the length between your right fingertips and your left sit bone (as in Fig. B).

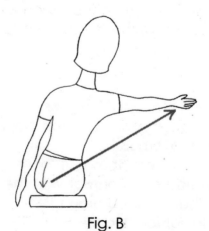

Fig. B

REACH FOR THE PHONE

Think of the arm movement coming from the whole of your back and not just from your right shoulder. You play out the movement like a measuring tape extending from a reel.

To return to the upright position, think of increasing the length of your right side, so that you rock back into the vertical position.

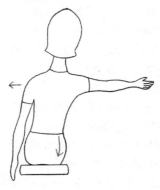

Important: do not pull on your left side and be careful not to let your dominant knee go in towards the centre line as you return to the upright position.

Repeat these movements, reaching to your left.

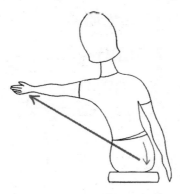

THE PRINCIPLE

When we reach for something it is easy to tense up and go for it. This is entirely counterproductive. By stopping and thinking, you enjoy the full, released length of your arms and your body remains relaxed, energised and your muscles retain their full suppleness and length.

Rock climbers understand this better than most. When balanced on a tiny foothold and stretching towards a handhold which seems at first to be out of reach, relaxing the shoulder allows the climber to gain the hold. Tightening up the shoulder, arm and hand would have the effect of shortening the climber's reach.

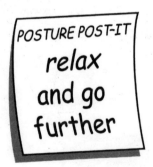

POSTURE POST-IT
*relax
and go
further*

REORGANISE YOUR LIFE

The obvious point of reorganisation is to put things within easy reach. But don't overdo this – put a few lightweight, regularly used items just out of reach as an excuse to try out the exercises above and let yourself enjoy the new feeling of being longer and leaner.

Finally, if you have to reach for something behind you, make sure that the whole of your body goes round with you. Do not try and twist the upper half of your body by tensing your knees and legs and corkscrewing your spine.

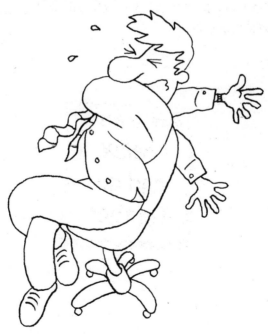

CHAPTER 8

LOOK LIVELY

THE PROBLEM

Boredom and monotony lead to sluggish vision and that in turn produces more monotony and boredom. It's a downward spiral. You might think that your stiff neck, fatigue, lack of energy and lethargy have nothing to do with the way you use your eyes. But you would be wrong! So, how do you use your eyes in such a way as to avoid these dismal states and choose instead to be lively and energetic?

THE EXERCISES

Exercise 1:

Stand and find an inanimate object at around eye level to focus on. Keeping focused on this object all the time, start moving your head around very slowly and in all sorts of movements, while keeping your feet where they are. For example, you might explore leaning your head backwards so that you are looking down the length of your nose as you drop back, bending your knees to stay balanced.

Or try turning as far as possible to the left, keeping your eyes on your chosen object.

Explore the number of movements you can make whilst maintaining eye contact with the object.

Exercise 2:

The previous exercise encourages your eyes to move. Now that your eyes are limbered up, try this simple exercise.

Sit and imagine that you are about to look at a picture on the wall behind you. Try miming this and notice how far your head goes round before your shoulders and torso start to move too. Now come back to your original position and look straight ahead. Imagine you are going to look at the picture behind you again, but this time let your eyes go all the way round before your head starts to move. Think of your eyes towing your head around. You will find that your head goes round much further than before.

As your head reaches its new finishing point, allow the rest of your torso to spiral after it in a lengthening movement from the sit bones and hips (which, if they are moving freely, means that you will be loose in your knee joints).

Now return – with your eyes leading – back to your original position.

Go through this again on the other side.

Exercise 3:
When sitting at your desk, focus on a point at eye level in front of you and allow yourself to become aware of your peripheral vision. Without moving your head or eyes, how much can you see to either side of you?

Whilst remaining focused on the point in front of you, think of lengthening your neck, allowing your head to roll forward and up, and become aware of how much farther your peripheral vision extends either side of you.

 THE PRINCIPLE

When we are in negative states – under pressure and anxious or under-stretched and bored, or worse still, both of these situations at the same time – we develop unhelpful and debilitating ways of dealing with them; we employ what might be called the 'don't ask' look, deliberately avoiding eye contact with others, keeping your eyes fixed and almost immobile.

Our eyes also become very tired when fixed for long periods of time on, for example, a computer screen. The exercises will help you address that problem, as they invite you to unfix your gaze and vary your focal length. Try to get into the habit of doing them from time to time during the day.

Related to this is another lost art, that of our eyes leading, as in Exercise 2. If you ask a child to look at a bird directly above them, that child's eyes will travel right up before any head movement occurs. Only then will the child's head tilt back.

We limit the freedom of our necks – and so all of our body – when we treat our eyes as though they are passive, unfocused passengers in our heads; if your eyes are open, they need to be alert and focused. If your eyes are not focused, you will feel progressively more tired and tense as the day goes on because part of you is not functioning as it should. And remember that focused eyes look more attractive.

One of the reasons holidays and excursions are so beneficial is that the novelty of that bit of scenery or that picture at an exhibition invites your eyes to focus and to stay focused.

Notice, by the way, in Exercise 3, how much more peripheral vision you have when you remember to release and lengthen your neck and think of that string taking you up from the crown of your head, as described in Chapter 3.

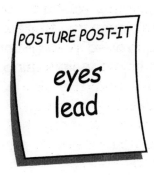

 REORGANISE YOUR LIFE

The way in which we look at the world will take us time to change. But the benefits are so great that it is worth thinking about how to re-organise to accommodate the exercises and change our visual habits. As for organising your time to go through the exercises, well, like all the exercises in this book, the more you can find time to perform them, the better. It is certainly true that you will obviously look as though you are performing exercises of some sort. Fine! Re-organise your attitude. You will find that anyone seen to be working on self-improvement is seen to be valuing themselves and that sends out a very potent message indeed. In addition to doing the exercises, try this: the next time you walk into your work place – or any place or situation that you feel is boringly familiar – talk yourself into focusing on the objects around you. See the sharpness of the edges, the colours, the shadows and shapes. Give everything around you the sort of attention you might give if you were seeing it for the first time.

CHAPTER 9

LYING DOWN – AND WORKING

THE PROBLEM

Chapter 4 explained the basic principle of lying in semi-supine, so if you have been practising this, you should by now be experiencing the benefits and may feel that you want to take this essential exercise a bit further. For example, you might feel that you could release your lower back more, or that your shoulders remain stubbornly nearer to your ears than the floor. All of the following exercises are performed in semi-supine and will help you to use your time spent in the position in an even more constructive way. But don't be in a rush to start these exercises: learning to lie still and be at rest is an art in itself and one that it is important to work at and re-acquire.

THE EXERCISES

Exercise 1:

Lie down in semi-supine. Bring your thoughts down the length of your body and focus them on your left leg. With your knees still bent, start to allow your left leg to waft gently outwards from your body, then back to where it started, and then inwards towards the other leg, all in a continuous, slow movement. Check on a number of things as you do this. Is the left side of your pelvis lifting off the floor as your knee moves inwards and over towards your other leg? If your leg is moving freely in the ball and socket joint of your hip, this will not happen. Is your left foot turning and lifting very early in the movement? If your shin is moving freely over your ankle, this will not happen. If you are moving freely, you will feel as if the top of your thigh is lengthening and easing your kneecap slightly further forward as you move your bent leg outwards and then again as you move it over towards your other knee. (If you are releasing the muscles of your inner thigh as you move you will find that this will happen naturally. It is another way in which you will know that you are allowing the movement, rather than forcing it.) Repeat this with the other leg.

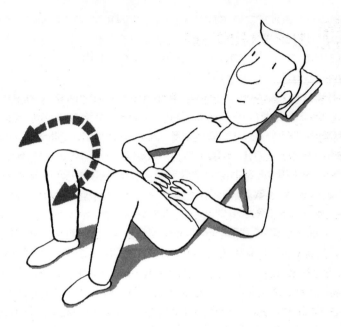

Exercise 2:

In semi-supine, once again think along the length of your spine and down into your right leg. Keeping your leg bent, bring it up towards your chest. First, perform this action as you would automatically, just bringing your leg up quite quickly, and observe how much your spine (which includes your neck) tightens and how much your body lifts and rocks away from the floor. At this point, most of us find that a considerable amount of extra, unnecessary movement is going on. Now try it a second time. This time work very hard with your mind and make much less effort with your body. Think along the length of your spine and out towards your right leg.

Before you begin, check that you haven't tightened your knee inwards in (mistaken) preparation for the movement. If you have tightened it, loosen and rebalance your knee. Imagine a length of string attached to your knee, drawing it easily and lightly towards your chest. Visualise the length of your back feeding into the underside of your leg, causing your whole leg to rise effortlessly. Your spine continues to be a stable, heavy weight in contact with the floor. Allow your leg to come towards your body as a baby's might; effortlessly and without strain. Take your time and refine the action of raising your leg until you can perform it without any of those extra tensions.

So far the exercise has involved stopping and thinking about the way you use your body in order to perform an ordinary movement with much less effort. You can go on to help your back still further in the following way: as your leg comes towards your body, interlace your fingers and let your arms float up to place your linked hands over your bent knee, as far down your shin as possible without strain (being especially aware of keeping your neck free of tension). At this point it is important to resist the urge to pull your knee towards your chest. Rather, allow the combined weight of your bent leg and relaxed arms, dropping down to the elbows, to gently ease tension out of your lower back. If you are patient and wait you will find that this happens simply and naturally.

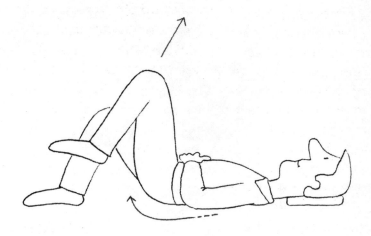

Exercise 3:

The two exercises above concern your lower body. The following exercise focuses on your upper body and will help you to free up your shoulders. As you are lying down in semi-supine, visualise a beach ball floating somewhere above your chest. Imagine it to be very light, full of helium. Then, let your arms float up to catch the ball. Now pretend you are examining every part of the ball: keep your hands the same width apart and rotate the joints of your wrists, elbows and shoulders through an extensive range of movements, as you would if you were rotating a ball on each of its axes. But do not do this for very long at a time: As soon as your arms feel tired, let the ball float away and your arms drop gently back onto your body again.

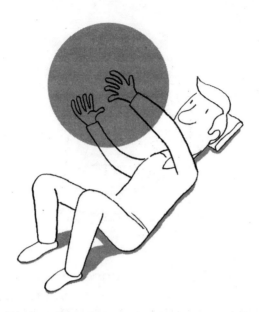

 THE PRINCIPLE

Working slowly and scrupulously you allow yourself time to monitor the unnecessary tensions which are involved in the simplest of actions. For example, Exercise 2 refers to the action of raising the leg as a baby might; easily and without effort. We are still able to perform that and many other actions in this simple, unhindered way. This, by the way, is preparation for walking. Although you are lying down, the relationship of your legs to your spine is the same, so by practising raising your leg you are also practising good walking, without your leg movement creating any lurching and pulling in your spine (see Chapter 10).

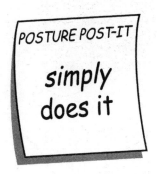

 REORGANISE YOUR LIFE

There is a temptation to rush into exercise. Take the time to settle into semi-supine for at least five minutes before you begin this work. Stop, identify what you're doing and reorganise the movement you're about to make. In an apparently passive situation, you are going to be working hard to reorganise your muscles to do things in a new and more relaxed way. Initially, if this feels easy, you are almost certainly doing it wrong!

CHAPTER 10

STANDING STILL AND GETTING ABOUT

THE PROBLEM

Standing well is difficult. Less obviously, so is walking well. When we stand in an unbalanced way, we invite lower backache, tired, heavy and often painful legs. Most of us say we feel better when moving about but the way that we are moving our limbs when getting about often promotes tension in the spine and we then carry this stress pattern into other activities such as sitting. (The reverse is also true of course. Sitting habits carry through to affect walking and standing. For a more in depth discussion of stress free sitting, see Chapter 5.) The exercises in this chapter are intended to help you regain stress-free standing and walking.

THE EXERCISES

Exercise 1:
Find a level, comfortable surface (a carpeted floor is ideal) near to a wall, which you will later need for support. You may prefer to remove your shoes for this exercise. Stand with your hands by your sides, feet about hip-width apart. Distribute your weight equally between your two feet, avoiding any tendency to lean into your dominant side. Take a moment to ensure that your knees feel relaxed – that is, not locked back or pulled in towards each other.

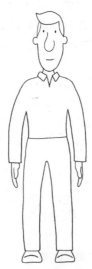

Allow your spine to lengthen, be aware of the balance of your head (remember the puppeteer; Chapter 3, Exercise 1) and allow your tailbone to drop. Let your hands drop to your sides with your thumbs pointing forwards.

Particularly notice where the weight of your body is referred down through your feet. If you are standing in a poised and balanced way, the weight is predominantly down through your heels and not the balls of your feet. It is distributed in a ratio of around 60 per cent through the heels and 40 per cent through the rest of your feet (excluding the arch). This may seem unfamiliar – you may feel as though you are falling backwards; this is most likely to be because you are used to putting too much weight onto your toes.

Notice if your pelvis is twisted. To check this, put your hands on the brim of your pelvis (what you might mistake for your hips) to monitor if one is more forward than the other.

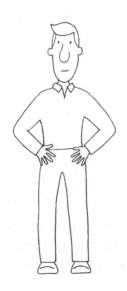

If this is the case, you are standing in a twisted position. Ease back on the side that was twisted forward until your torso is straightened.

Spread your hands and place the palms on the small of your back and ease back into them. As you release middle back tension you will find that your spine lengthens and your ribs drop down in front.

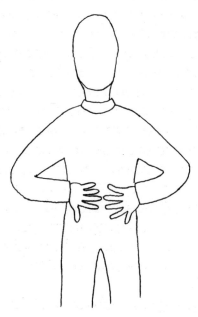

Let your arms drop by your sides again, thumbs forward. Now you are standing comfortably, we can begin.

Position yourself at right angles to the wall and about a foot away from it. Bring a hand up to rest on the wall to support you and rock back on your heels so that you are now standing on your heels only. In order to look at your feet, hinge forward very slightly at your hips (check the location of these in Body Map) maintaining the length of your head, neck and back. Now, very scrupulously and as slowly as you are able, replace both your feet on the floor simultaneously, finding first the outer borders and then the little toes and then other toes and finally your big toe. At this moment, when your big toe is comfortably in contact with the floor, *stop*. It is likely that you will be tempted with one or both of your feet to go that little bit too far at the end of the movement. If you are pulling your knees together, you will be pressing down on the arch of one or both of your feet. If this was even slightly the case, repeat the exercise both now and from time to time in the future until you can quite easily resist the impulse to go too far. It might help you, by the way, to think what sort of footprint your feet would make if you were bringing them down onto warm, wet sand. A perfect footprint would *not* show the imprint of the arch of your foot. Now you are ready to start moving.

You are going to monitor the movements you make as you practise some exaggerated walking on the spot. Apart from keeping your head balanced and back long, do not worry too much about exactly how you walk on the spot. Take it slowly and bring your knees higher than you do when walking normally.

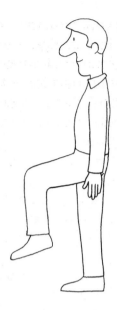

Notice two things:

– Whether there is any forward lurch of your spine with each leg lift; there should be gentle muscle movement and lengthening, but no lurching.

– How much your knees tense in towards each other at the start of each leg lift. They should not pull in at all.

Once you are happy that you've achieved these two objectives, it is time to move on to the next exercise.

Exercise 2:
Once again, begin by standing as before, poised and balanced, hands by your sides. Think about taking a step but don't move yet. When you do move it will be very slowly.

Without moving your torso forwards at all, shift your weight slightly onto your right foot and place your left foot on the ground in front of you. If your chin, neck or torso has leaned forwards to accomplish this – or worse still, all three – start again. Your foot starts the movement, not your chin or pelvis.

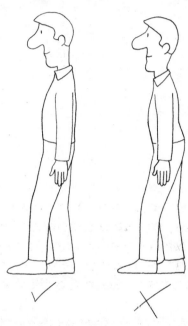

Your body weight stays back on your right foot. Lift the heel of your right foot and as you do so, feel your body being lifted and moved forward so that the weight comes to rest on your left foot. Your right foot is impelling you forward in a smooth, rocking movement. Feel your right foot being pleasantly worked as it lifts and rolls you up, forward and down.

Now your weight is entirely on your left foot. Move forward again by placing your right foot in front of your left, lift your left heel and transfer the weight to your right foot. Remember to only allow your torso forwards with the movement, not ahead of it.

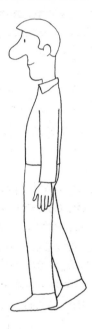

Now you are off and walking very slowly but with poise. It may feel odd but this is a slow-motion version of good walking. When you feel comfortable with this, gradually increase your pace to your normal walking speed.

Exercise 3:
This is an observational exercise which helps to clarify some of the principles in Exercise 2.

Find a clear, safe space in which to walk backwards. Begin by standing as before, hands by sides, looking straight ahead. Walk backwards at whatever pace makes you feel secure and comfortable. Then decide to walk forwards, changing direction in as smooth and uninterrupted a fashion as possible. As you walk forwards, take with you the positive feelings that walking backwards promoted; weight more back on your heels, a finer sense of balance (especially with regard to your head balanced on your spine – your head, neck and spine operating as one unit).

Two things to notice:
– You will see your feet moving on the lower edge of your peripheral vision as you walk forwards in a way that you can't if your chin and chest are being thrust out ahead of your feet. Seeing your feet in this way is a good indicator that your walking is becoming less of an effort and less thrusting – the precise opposite of the chin up and chest out approach.
– Secondly, be conscious of where the weight of your body is coming down through your feet. When you move in a more tension-free manner, you will feel more of the outside of your feet as you walk.

Exercise 4:
Stand as before and place your right foot in front of you. Transfer your weight evenly between your feet by bending your right knee slightly. The left leg stays

straight. The weight in each foot is predominantly down through the heel.

Your torso is balanced between your two feet and your body is facing forwards, not twisted at all.

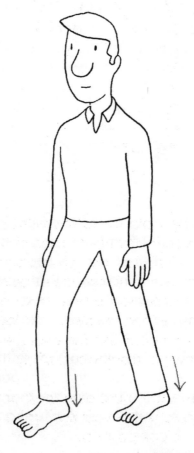

Start to move your right knee and lower leg in a slow, thoughtful, clockwise circle, pivoting around your ankle, exploring the full mobility of your joints.

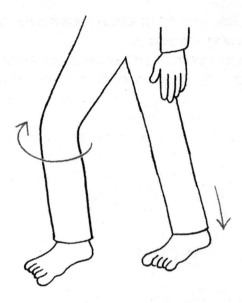

You should be able to do this without lifting your right big toe on the farthest reach of the circle.

If your toe is lifting off the ground on the outward rotation, stop and think what muscles you need to release in order to be able to accomplish it. Is there resistance in your knee, your lower back, or tension in your neck? Use the exercise as a way of exploring how your balanced body can be more flexible.

You may feel the muscles in the back of your left leg being stretched as your right knee approaches the twelve o'clock position.

Be aware of any tendency to press down on the arch of your left foot. If this is happening, your left knee is tending towards the centre line of your body. Keep it directed away.

Now take your right knee around again in an anticlockwise direction and explore how much movement is available on the inward rotation, without crushing down on the arch of your right foot. As you work, imagine you are on a beach and making a perfect footprint in the sand. Now bring your foot back and be amazed at how different it feels. In a very few minutes, working slowly with your mind engaged, a very simple exercise like this can be incredibly productive.

Now work the other foot in the same manner.

 THE PRINCIPLE

Standing still (Exercise 1) is an art that we need to re-learn. Our legs aren't meant to be stood upon for extended lengths of time, but sometimes we have to stand for longer than is good for us. We can look after ourselves and feel much lighter and freer by remembering to think of an imaginary string pulling the crown of our head upwards, and by not standing on the balls of our feet, but rather finding, as we release our necks, that the weight of our standing body is predominantly down through our heels and around the outer borders of our feet. Only then will our knees be unlocked – which allows our lower backs to be free of pain-inducing tension.

As for walking, even in a sedentary job we may take thousands of steps a day, and may take them in an effortful manner that puts stress on the spine.

The first two exercises focus on a common mistake in walking: moving the spine towards the leg rather than vice versa. In poised, balanced walking, your spine is carried along effortlessly. Think of length coming out of your back and travelling along the underside of your thigh and your walking will feel buoyant and light.

The third exercise demonstrates how you can move without strain. In walking backwards you are doing something that you so rarely do, that you will not have had the chance to learn and incorporate any damaging habits. The experience of feeling your body move in an unfamiliar, habit-free way helps you to map these sensations onto your usual walking action.

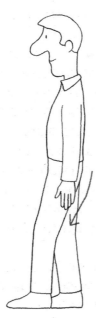

Exercise 4 recognises how much we restrict the flexibility of our lower limbs, unconsciously limiting the lateral movement of our knees and tightening our ankles. This exercise offers a way of regaining that flexibility.

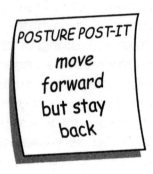

POSTURE POST-IT

move
forward
but stay
back

 REORGANISE YOUR LIFE

Make friends with your feet – they are doing an important job so trust them more. You wouldn't spend all day wearing gloves, and yet we often spend most of our waking hours wearing shoes. Give your feet a break – go shoeless when you can. Five minutes padding about barefoot on a carpeted floor can do wonders for recharging your energy levels.

Vary your shoes as often as possible; keep a separate pair at the office and a different pair for driving. When buying shoes, think about giving your feet some breathing space. Your upright body balances through your feet; by allowing them to be as unconstricted as possible, your whole sense of balance will improve.

Incidentally, your legs are not meant for standing. They are a delicate system of levers for moving us around the planet. The tonic quality of the muscles is lost if you use them as solid pillars for supporting your body when standing still. Keep moving over your ankles, if only very slightly – do not let your legs become fixed and locked.

Be careful carrying a bag over your shoulder; not only may you find that you are hitching your shoulder up, but if the bag is bulky you may be walking and standing in a twisted way to accommodate it. If so, reorganise by wearing it more centrally, to the front or back of your body or invest in a new bag.

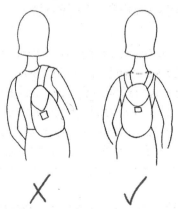

The things we wear and carry are not supposed to damage us!

CHAPTER 11

THE WORLD ON YOUR SHOULDERS

THE PROBLEM

Most of us go around with our shoulders tensed for the majority of the time, usually without realising it.

As you become more tense, your shoulders creep closer to your ears, your neck tenses up and your shoulders and chest narrow, and this constricts how easily you breathe. Your shoulders are doing more work than they need to and you feel more tired as a consequence.

Shoulder tension is also a significant contributor to some forms of repetitive strain injury. And remember: tense shoulders not only make you feel bad, they make you look bad; less confident and less assertive. The secret isn't to walk around in a parade ground posture, but to find a way to relax the shoulders and stop them wasting so much of your energy.

THE EXERCISES

Exercise 1:

A really easy exercise to begin.

Sit down with your hands on your knees, palms down. Think about the balance of your head on your neck (see Chapter 3, Exercise 1). Now, slowly rotate your hands outwards until they are resting palms upwards. Notice how this widens you across the top of the chest.

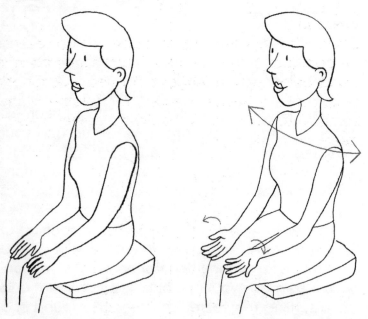

Now stand. As your arms drop by your sides, allow your hands to rotate outwards slightly until your thumbs are forwards.

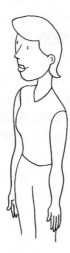

Exercise 2:

Stand with your feet slightly apart, weight evenly on both feet, hands by sides, thumbs forward and head balanced on lengthening neck. Gradually bring your left shoulder and left ear together at the same time. Make sure your other shoulder doesn't move in the meantime.

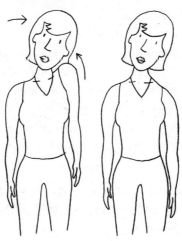

With your head still on one side, let your left arm and shoulder drop down the side of your body as far as you can.

Notice how far down the length of your body your hand has been allowed to drop. Leaving your arm and shoulder in their new, relaxed length, only now restore your head to the upright position.

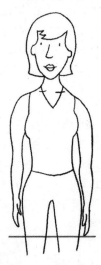

Continue the exercise with the right side, this time making sure that your left shoulder doesn't move. As you do this exercise, you may feel your shoulders and neck being stretched. This is good. We're so familiar with the feeling of shoulders being high we don't notice it, so this exercise is a habit-breaker.

Repeat the exercise at regular intervals and as you feel you need it. Start earlier in the day and catch yourself before you start the old familiar tension-filled routine.

Exercise 3:

For this exercise, ideally you will enlist a friend to observe you.

Stand up with your arms dropping by your sides, hands relaxed. Rotate your hands so that your thumbs point forwards and you feel your elbows rotating further into your sides. Relax your shoulders and allow your arms to be their true length (as in Exercise 2). Move your right arm very slowly sideways, away from your body, stopping the minute you (or your friend) observe that your right shoulder is rising.

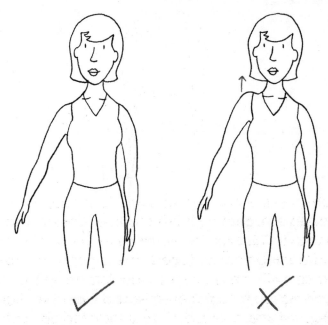

Allow the underside of your arm to lengthen as though a friendly puppeteer is taking your arm out through strings on the fingertips.

Let your arm come out at right angles to your body (it may tend to move forwards but think of it drifting back into place).

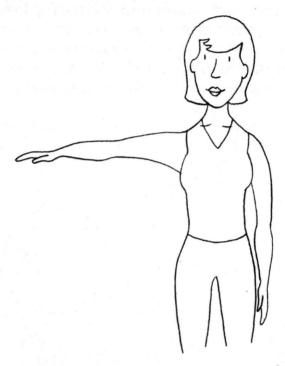

This is very gentle, but what you are doing is radically changing the way you use your body. You're using your shoulder as a lever, not a hoist. You can expect to feel quite a pull and maybe some discomfort at first, particularly on the underused underside of your arm. Now continue the exercise by working with the other arm.

This exercise can be extended in the following way:

Take your hand outwards until it is around 30 cm from your body. Then rotate your hand at the wrist until the palm is facing forwards. Let your shoulder drop and, with your hand still facing forwards, bring your arm behind your back, as though you are about to pat yourself just below your bottom. (If you are patting yourself on the bottom, your shoulder and arm are not relaxed enough.)

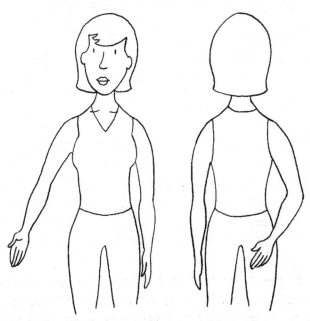

Rotate your hand again at the wrist, so the back of your hand is against your body. Hinge at the elbow and start to move your hand and forearm up your back, as though feeling for a zip. Move as far as you can and then relax and drop your elbow and shoulder.

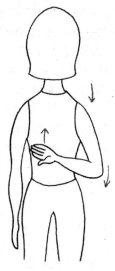

This will, in the short term, move your arm further down your back. However, if you proceed in this way, constantly relaxing and dropping your elbow and shoulder and then moving up again you will find that you will actually, ultimately, reach much higher than you were able to before.

Now continue this exercise with the other arm.

As you get used to the feel of these exercises, you'll learn to involve your shoulders less in everyday movements. You'll relax more across the top of your arms and shoulders and your arms will regain their natural length.

 THE PRINCIPLE

Most of the activities we perform are performed over and over again in the same situation – at a desk, at a drawing board, at the kitchen sink. We allow ourselves to become drawn into whatever it is that we are working on. Our shoulders become rounded, our chests narrow – we can be a good two shirt or blouse sizes narrower than we need be – and our shoulders creep higher. Not only are your shoulders up around your ears but the whole of the upper torso is narrower because your chest and back muscles are all contracting in towards the centre. After a while this misuse becomes familiar and habitual.

What's more, we don't look good. Because we have narrowed our upper torso, we look less assertive. When the shoulders are hunched, the pectoral or chest muscles are shortened, which makes the whole of the torso looks narrower. When we are tense and the muscles are contracted – the effect is as though a fan has closed. When the shoulder and chest muscles release, they lengthen and you look wider across the top of your chest and shoulders. The fan has opened into its natural state.

These exercises help us to unlearn shoulder tension. Moving the arms sideways, as in Exercise 3, gets us used to the idea of lengthening the muscles on the underside of our arms instead of using our shoulders to lift our hands. This is particularly important when sitting at a desk, lifting the hands to begin to type, write or draw; the unhelpful habit of tightening hands, wrists and arms establishes just the right muscular environment to encourage repetitive strain injury!

Releasing and dropping your shoulder and elbow when performing arm actions may seem counter-intuitive, but you reach much farther by doing so and you are maintaining your arm's true length and the tonic quality of your muscles. You are also able to perform actions which you might have previously given up on, just because you were performing them in a tight, impatient and tense way. For more on this, see Chapter 7.

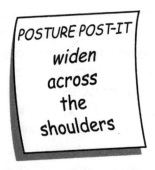

POSTURE POST-IT
widen
across
the
shoulders

 REORGANISE YOUR LIFE

Make your environment feel as if it's your own space. Be in control of your own territory and everything in it; screens, plants, shelves, even photographs. This will help you feel more open, positive and relaxed.

Before you do any work at a desk, stop and think of relaxing those shoulders and lengthening the underside of your arm. Concert pianists can sit for a long period before raising their hands to the keyboard. Part of this is to reorganise the body to perform. Think particularly of letting weight drop into the points of your elbows before moving your hands on top of the keyboard, and let your arms hinge easily at the elbow without any pulling up to the shoulder.

Most office activities can be used as an excuse to work on yourself, ridding yourself of damaging habits. When using the telephone, for example, bring the phone to your ear, not your ear to the phone, and be aware of the balance of your head on the top of your neck, shoulders relaxed. And remember, when carrying anything, as far as possible make sure the weight is equally divided between your two arms.

CHAPTER 12

FLEXIBLE FRIENDS

THE PROBLEM

Not feeling so mobile in your hands and wrists these days? Do they feel aching and stiff, especially in the morning? And do you feel increasing discomfort in your upper limbs? This could be the onset of repetitive strain injury. It certainly signals a need to keep your joints flexible, especially if your work requires repeated actions e.g. computer typing, playing an instrument, working at a desk; all of these mean we are using our hands and arms in a repetitive way. Many tasks use a very limited range of movement, and the more limited the more potentially damaging. We can't or don't want to change our jobs, so what can we do to help to keep ourselves flexible?

THE EXERCISES

Exercise 1:

Standing or sitting, think of your spine lengthening and shoulders and elbows dropping as you hold your hands in front of you, arms bent at the elbow. Begin with palms facing each other.

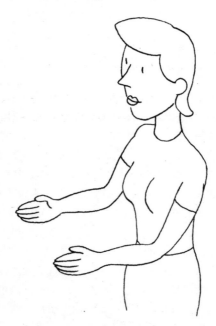

Pretend that you have got water on your hands and shake them from side to side to dry them, keeping your wrists relaxed. Don't shake too hard – use the weight of your hands to explore the limits of movement you have in your wrists. Keep the palms facing each other throughout this exercise.

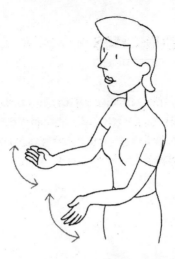

Then turn your hands palm downwards and shake them again, this time in a vertical direction.

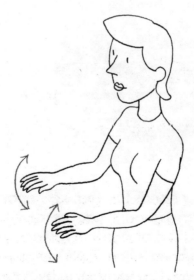

Then repeat the first movement, with palms facing.

Exercise 2:
(This is a slightly different version of the beach ball exercise described in Chapter 9.) Sitting or standing as in Exercise 1, hold your hands in front of you, palms facing each other. Imagine you have a large, lightweight beach ball between your hands (the beach ball's diameter is the same as the width across your chest).

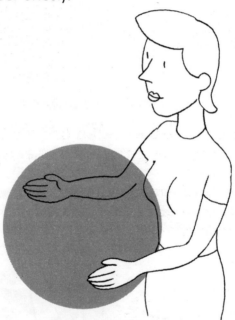

Keeping your hands the same distance apart, start to move them as though you are rotating the beach ball, first rotating about the vertical axis, then the horizontal one – as if the ball's surface is covered in writing and you are examining every word.

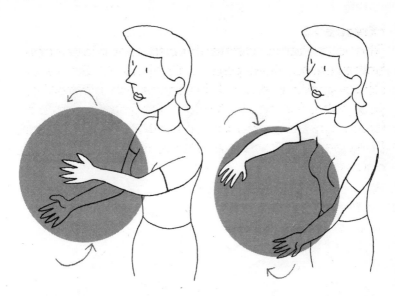

This will take your elbows, wrists and the ball and socket joint of your arms into some previously unvisited places!

Keep the three-dimensional image of the ball strong in your mind so that your palms stay the same distance apart.

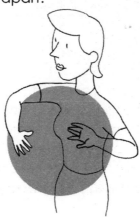

Exercise 3:
Standing, bring one hand up in front of you, palm facing away from you.

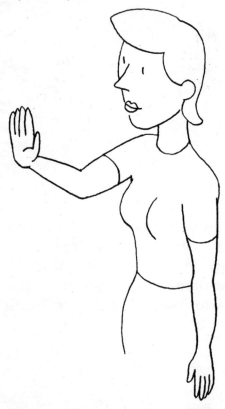

Imagine standing in front of a shop window. Your hand is going to wipe along the width of it.

Start to move your hand along the glass, away from the centre of your body. Keep the image strong – the palm of your hand is going to continue along the glass, as if you are cleaning it with a smooth cloth.

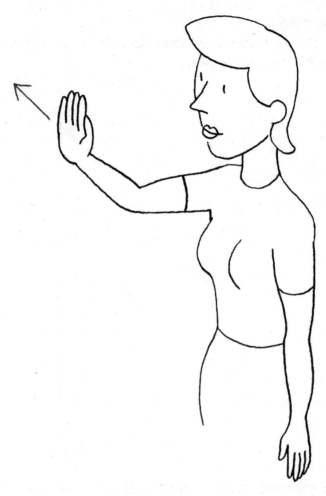

Do not allow your shoulder to rise as your hand moves away from you. When you feel you are approaching the limit of your movement, relax (and drop) your shoulder to allow more length in the underside of your upper arm, which in turn allows your hand to extend a few centimetres farther.

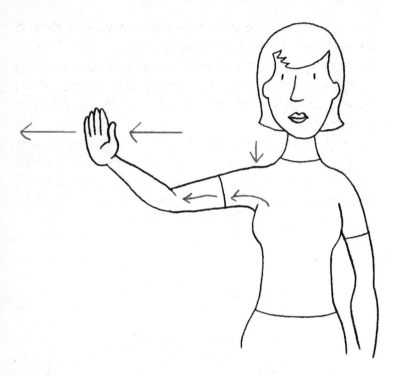

Don't expect to be able to reach too much farther, especially on the first attempt. It is the final part of the exercise which is important and you will find you can extend your hand a little farther each time. The length is achieved by dropping your shoulder and not by leaning outwards.

 THE PRINCIPLE

Performing the opposite move to the one you keep repeating all the time promotes mobility and extends underused muscles. Over time, when you are performing repetitive actions day after day, a limited set of muscles may be used. The mobility of your joints can become restricted, resulting in stiffness and pain. The immobility comes from overusing one set of muscles and underusing others.

Bringing your awareness into these areas and exploring their natural range of movement helps keep them flexible. To do this, you need to take the movement to its limit (not below it) in a carefully monitored fashion. Do not overdo it.

POSTURE POST-IT

*explore
all the
parts*

REORGANISE YOUR LIFE

Ask yourself where your joints have not moved to today. Look at how you perform repetitive actions. What are the opposite actions? Can you identify the underused muscles? If so, give them a brief workout and give those overused muscles a holiday.

As well as the exercises above, find time to explore one joint per day. For example, Wednesday is elbow day. Really get to know how flexible this marvel of natural engineering can be. Release the muscles and remember to allow your spine, shoulder and arms to lengthen as you move and explore your joints.

CHAPTER 13

LIFT OFF

THE PROBLEM

Lifting anything – whether heavy or not – is a health and safety issue. You may already have suffered the consequences of lifting inappropriately; backache, muscle spasms, a slipped disc. In this chapter we will look at lifting objects, including the way that you do so when the only object you have to lift is yourself.

THE EXERCISES

Exercise 1:

This exercise will help you learn to bend and straighten without tightening your lower back.

Find a clear wall and stand with your feet five to eight centimetres from it. Lean back so that the wall supports you. Your feet should be hip-width apart, hands dropping by your sides, head balanced and neck lengthening (but both head and neck clear of the wall).

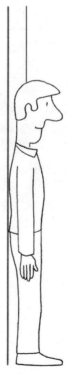

Lower yourself down the wall into a shallow squat – you will not be descending very far, perhaps 10 cm at most. Think of your knees gently buckling to allow you to slide down the wall. Do not force anything. The weight of your body should be mainly down through your heels.

If you find your back is losing contact with the wall, it is because you are tensing your lower back and arching your spine. If this happens, halt your descent, release the tension and lean back into the wall before continuing.

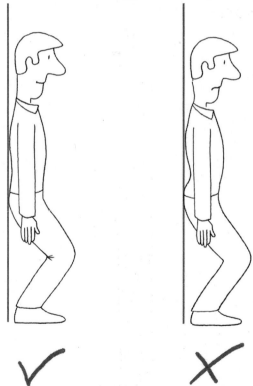

Come to a halt and, as slowly as possible, reverse the move. The weight of your body should again be in your heels. Be aware of your contact with the wall. You are using the wall as a reference point to check if your lower back is tensing as you bring yourself back into a fully standing position. Especially at the last moment – as you are about to stand fully – use the wall to help you resist the temptation to tighten and arch away from the wall. Keep your back in contact with the wall. This may cause your legs to tremble slightly, but as you get used to standing without tensing, the trembling will cease.

Exercise 2:

Find a flight of stairs where you can work on this exercise undisturbed. Stand at the foot of the stairs. Think of a string taking the crown of your head upwards.

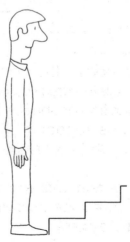

Feel the weight of your body principally through your heels. Shift your weight slightly to transfer it onto your left leg. Keeping your head balanced, neck and back aligned, and without any forward lurch of your spine, bring your right foot up and place it on the first step.

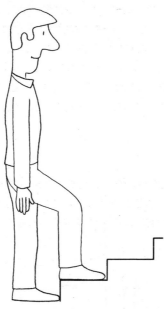

This is the critical point – the start of the action. If your right knee pulls inwards as you bring your foot up, this is an indication of unnecessary tension and effort. In which case, repeat the action, thinking of releasing the tension in your upper leg as you lift your foot.

(Practising this action until you can lift your foot without tensing your knee inwards is beneficial in itself. It is a habit-breaker.)

Place your foot – the whole length of your foot, not just the ball of your foot – onto the stair. Take a step upwards with the weight of your body going down principally through your right heel. (If the tread of the stairway is too narrow to allow this, find another staircase.)

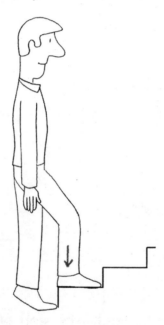

Continue up the staircase being conscious of:
– the imaginary string taking you upwards from the crown of your head
– weight going down through your heels
– your knees drifting outwards from the centre line of your body.
Coming down again:
Avoid the mistake of thrusting your head and

neck forwards in order to look at the stairs. Instead, hinge forwards slightly from the hips.

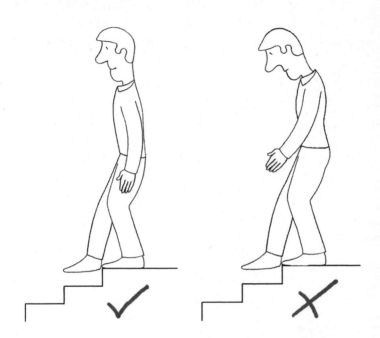

Toes and then heel contact each step as you lower yourself downstairs. Keep in mind that your weight goes mainly down through your heels and keep thinking up (remember the imaginary string on the crown of your head). Don't forget those knees drifting away from each other.

Progress seems slow at first but your posture is very secure and you will be doing far less work as a result.

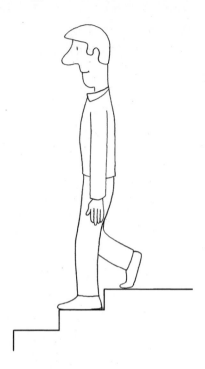

Exercise 3:
Take two books and place one of them on the floor.
Place the other on the seat of a chair so that it is just
below your reach. Approach the book on the floor
and stand as close as possible – we usually stand
too far away from the object we are going to pick
up. Place your feet farther apart – you will almost
certainly have instinctively stood with your feet too
close together. You don't have to square up to the
book, the most important factor is to keep a good
distance between your heels.

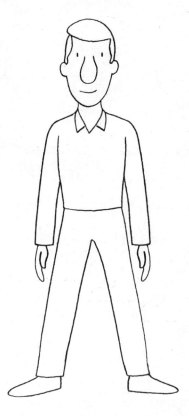

Think of the imaginary string from the crown of your head keeping your head balanced and neck long, then begin to go into a squat. Make sure that you keep your feet fully in contact with the floor, the weight of your body dropping down through your heels and not transferring too much onto your toes. If, as you squat, your heels come off the ground, your feet are probably too close together. Move them farther apart and start again. If you are wearing shoes with pronounced heels, take them off.

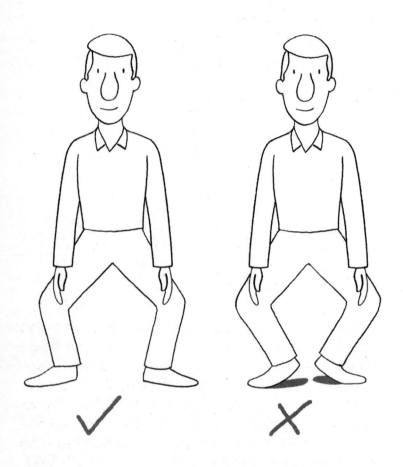

As you descend, pivot your body slightly at the hips to allow you to reach forwards between your knees and pick up the book. Your weight should always remain principally down through your heels and the weight of your back should fall behind the line of your hips.

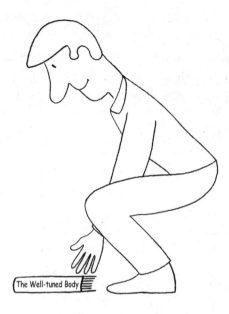

The Well-tuned Body

Pick up the book and reverse the action to stand up: think of the string on the crown of your head taking you up, and your weight moving down through your heels and not forward onto your toes. As you straighten your legs, think of your tailbone dropping, as you practised in Exercise 1. Your head, neck and back stay relaxed and lengthening throughout.

Now for the second book. In many ways this is trickier because of our preconceptions; it requires you to make a revised visual judgement as to how you perform the action.

Once you have gauged that the book is out of reach – however marginally – perform a mini-squat to lower your body and enable yourself to pick up the book. This way, you are using your legs to do the work and keeping your spine free from unnecessary tension. It avoids the maladroit regime of a jutting-out chin, bending from the waist and legs held stiffly to keep you balanced, which is potentially damaging and looks ungainly.

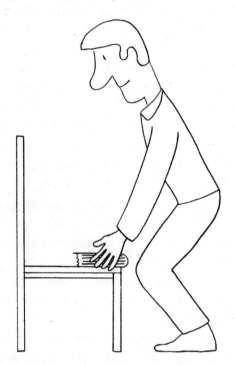

 THE PRINCIPLE

Heels down, knees away from each other.

If you have been following the chapters of this book in sequence, you will find these ideas familiar by now. When you are lifting anything, including your own body, your legs do the work. If you become unbalanced through your weight being too far forward onto your toes, your lower back is likely to go into spasm to protect itself as it is made to perform an action that is potentially damaging.

When standing up, tightening the lower back is such a compulsive habit that most of us are not even aware when we are doing it. Exercise 1 helps us to become aware of what we are doing to ourselves and to relearn an apparently simple action. We are also reminding ourselves that lifting does not just involve other objects – it also means ourselves. See Chapter 6 for more on this.

In Exercise 2, we find that if we are trying to lift ourselves through our toes, our legs are bound to tighten. The result is that our back will also be tense. There is no need for this – the action can be undertaken in a much less stressful and less energy-wasting fashion. The exercise also demonstrates that poised movements feel more secure. We could stop at any moment in this exercise without feeling off-balance.

Exercise 3 encourages you to use that funny pair of hinges halfway up your legs. Use those knees! It also highlights the danger that the nearer the object, the more likely you are to take potentially damaging short cuts. This applies to any activity which involves losing height. Squatting into such tasks is not only more efficient, it also keeps your hips mobile. Many people become stiff in their hips partly because they keep their legs tense instead of using their knees when bending.

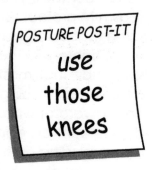

 REORGANISE YOUR LIFE

Most of us have evolved complicated sets of habits around everyday activities. Bending and straightening actions are probably the most revealing of these habits. People do not use their knees enough! Keep this in mind when approaching even apparently innocuous activities such as taking a book or goods from the lower shelves of the library or supermarket. It may seem strange at first but it is more natural and graceful to do a semi squat rather than a bend from the waist.

Every change of height is an opportunity to practise keeping yourself flexible.

CHAPTER 14

DON'T HOLD YOUR BREATH

THE PROBLEM

If you find yourself suffering from breathlessness or fatigue, feelings of remoteness, light headedness or poor circulation, it may be a sign that you have acquired bad breathing habits. How do we re-learn good breathing? First, your breathing is affected by whatever else is happening to your body, for example, if your are sitting hunched over a desk. So the first step to better breathing is to follow the advice contained in the earlier chapters of this book. This chapter gives you a specific exercise to help you regain natural breathing.

THE EXERCISE

You can work on this exercise either sitting or lying down. Lying in a semi-supine position (see Chapter 4) is ideal because the intercostals (the muscles between your ribs) are potentially at their most relaxed in this position.

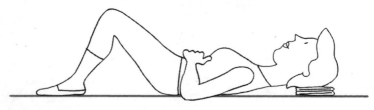

Start by thinking of lengthening and widening your body. Become aware of your breathing; don't be judgemental about it, you're observing, not getting self-critical. Do not try to alter anything, although you may find your breathing changes for the better simply due to this self-monitoring. Focus more on the out breath than the in breath, as though exhaling is full of subtlety and interest. Notice how it varies from one breath to another – the length of each one, for example. This may cause your breath to naturally slow down. Be aware that it is natural to pause briefly between the out breath and the in breath. Respect the pause and do not rush into the in breath, otherwise you risk hyperventilation.

After a few minutes of observation, begin enhancing the out breath by adding a whispered sound, the sound 'ahh'. Let the sound escape through slightly parted lips, almost like a sigh – you are letting go of the breath, not forcing it out; think of the contrast between letting air out of a balloon and the effort of blowing it up.

Think of your out breath as having length; imagine your breath moving along the whole length of your spine.

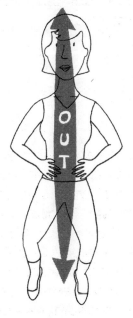

After half a dozen whispered 'ahh' sounds, turn your attention to your in breath. It will already be more natural and efficient as a result of your more complete out breath, but enhance it further by noticing your ribs (the complete span, including the ribs in your back and sides) moving out towards your elbows, like sails caught in the wind. Again, you are allowing this to happen and not forcing anything.

Imagine your in breath as having width, travelling easily through the breadth of your body.

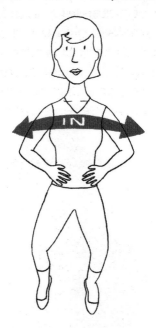

Out is long, in is wide. Let go on the out breath, clearing the lungs of old air, leaving room for reviving air on the in breath. Think of letting go of stressful, negative thoughts as you let the breath go out – let them float away on the whispered 'ahh'.

 THE PRINCIPLE

We under-breathe in times of stress and develop bad breathing habits. For example, when we concentrate we tend to hold our breath. We under-breathe when people invade our space.

Paradoxically, smokers often under-breathe when not smoking because they have started to rely on the exhalation of cigarette smoke in order to fully exhale. When smokers give up, they often find it hard to get back to natural breathing.

It is not useful to 'take a deep breath' – that just promotes more tension. 'Chin up, chest out, take a deep breath' is the very reverse of natural breathing.

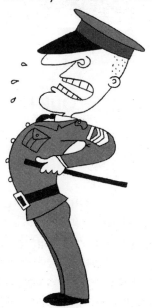

The 'ahh' sound raises the soft palate (the softer part of your upper mouth) and helps free the airways. This breathing practice is not something you do all the time but it helps retrain your body to breathe more fully and naturally, working against the ingrained habit of under-breathing. It stimulates your body to better everyday use.

POSTURE POST-IT
*let go
with the
out breath*

 REORGANISE YOUR LIFE

Smell your environment. Are you not breathing fully because you don't want to? Bad air days need strategy; nice smells (oils, plants, flowers), ionisers, or reminders of better atmospheres (photographs of the seaside or the countryside).

If you do find that you are in a situation where your space is invaded (crushed on the tube or in a lift) and you feel deprived of oxygen, don't hold your breath or take shallow breaths; focus on breathing more completely and make the best of every out breath to rid yourself of inhaled toxins and stale air.

CHAPTER 15

PAIRING UP

THE PROBLEM

In everyday life, it is hard to stay in the moment and not anticipate your next physical movement all the time. When problems build up, the last thing we think about is our own sense of body awareness. These exercises help address that problem with the aid of a willing partner. If possible, try to find a partner who is around the same height as you for these exercises.

THE EXERCISES

Exercise 1:

Your partner is seated on a stool (see Chapter 5), eyes closed, shoes removed, with enough space for you to walk comfortably around them. Start touching your partner on the joints of their hands and feet, knees, neck and shoulders, and along what you can identify of their spine. Using only your middle finger, and alternating between your left and right middle fingers, this touch needs to be brief and gentle, as though you are transferring a drop of water from your fingertip onto your partner's body. Work precisely and attentively, and try to make contact with as many of your partner's joints as possible, but do this *slowly*, leaving at least five seconds between each contact. Make it random: for example, you might touch your partner's right shoulder and then the next time their left little toe. Your partner should experience this as a very gentle contact. (If not, it may be that you need to pay more attention to your own body use!)

This is very like the mental exercise in Chapter 4, in the sense that it encourages you to focus on specific points of your body at a time. After around ten minutes, change places; you take the stool, close your eyes and let your partner scatter the raindrops. Bizarre as this might sound, you are almost certain to find it extremely relaxing.

Exercise 2:
Stand and face your partner, about a foot apart. Think about how you are standing, as in Chapter 10, Exercise 1. Bring your right hand up in the space between you, palm outwards, about as high as your partner's chest. Your partner should then bring their left hand up, palm outwards, to meet yours and make palm-to-palm contact. Now ease your palms away from each other, transferring the contact to your fingertips, so that only your fingertips are touching. Imagine that your fingers are so sticky that the contact makes them stick together. Begin to move your right hand and arm and, as you do so, your partner should follow your movements, as if your fingers are 'stuck' together. Make the movement slow enough for your partner to keep the contact, increasing speed and range of movement as you sense it is possible to do this without losing that contact. So, you might start off with small, circular movements and then go on to larger, more random, and certainly less predictable ones.

After about three minutes, change over and start again, this time with your partner leading with their right hand and you following with your left hand. Complete the exercise by each taking a turn at leading with your left hand. Compare how much looser you both feel in your arms, wrists and shoulders after this exercise.

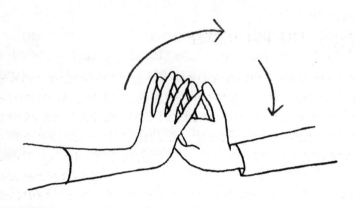

Exercise 3:

Sit facing your partner, close enough for you to touch hands. Now shut your eyes while your partner moves to interlink their hands and fingers to form a shape, for example, a butterfly or a rabbit (as if making a shadow picture on the wall) and then holds this position. Once your partner gives you the verbal signal that they have done this, keep your eyes closed and trace with your fingers your partner's hands and fingers, until you feel you have enough information to reproduce the shape they are making with your own hands and fingers. Your partner keeps their hands in their chosen shape while you do so. Keep your eyes shut, and only open them when you are satisfied that you have copied your partner's shape as nearly as possible. See how accurately (or otherwise!) you have made a copy. Swap roles, so that you make a shape with your hands and your partner copies it with their eyes closed.

THE PRINCIPLE

In Exercise 1, when you are the partner receiving the raindrops, the very randomness of the sequence invites you to settle back and not anticipate where your partner will touch you next. If your partner is working attentively, you will also feel that your whole body is being mapped out for your awareness through this gentle touch stimulation. In Exercise 2, when you are the one following your partner's movements, again the very random nature invites your muscles to cease predicting – the only way to follow is to stay with the movement and not think where you are going next. Exercise 3 speaks directly to your kinaesthetic sense – a necessary re-awakening for any body work.

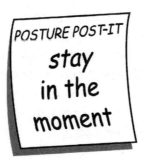

REORGANISE YOUR LIFE

These exercises will help you to reorganise your attitude to everyday movements. Instead of living in your head, or residing a few moments in the future as you anticipate what you are about to do next, take the time to focus on NOW.

CHAPTER 16

EVERY DAY IN EVERY WAY

THE PROBLEM

You have read the book, done the exercises and absorbed the principles. But what happens when you go out into the big wide world? In this chapter we will be looking at some everyday situations in order to see how you can pull all these ideas together. Alexander, in his work, observed that there are key areas of our bodies which are most commonly and habitually misused – the most important of these being the junction of the top of our spines with our heads (Chapter 3). But he made other observations too, and these form the basis for the suggestions, tips and hints in this book, summed up by the Posture Post-its.

Remember, the situations we are about to describe are only examples. The principles in the book apply to all activity, every day. They are a means of re-educating one's body to a new way of being.

1. IN THE RESTAURANT

Next time you are in a restaurant or café, or anywhere people are eating and drinking, look around you. What do you see? Most people will be making the mistake of being drawn into what they are doing, so that they are moving towards their food by bending their spines and sticking their chins out. Often they only have to lift their fork a short way to reach their mouth, so near are they to their plate.

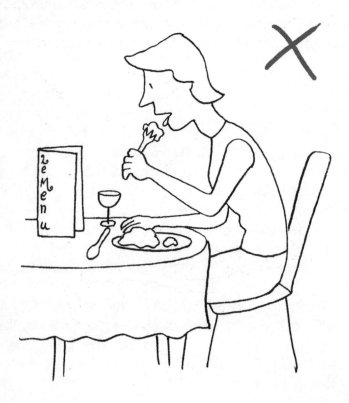

Think of it like this: there is the food in front of you and you are now going to reorganise the way you eat, just as you have learnt to reorganise the way you go forward to type, write or read (as detailed in Chapter 6). Keep your head, neck and back working as one unit as you hinge forward at your hips, just a sufficient amount to bring you to a comfortable angle over your food. Your legs and knees should stay relaxed and balanced. As you pick up your fork to eat, remain wide and open across the top of your body, shoulders and arms relaxed, as you hinge at the elbow to bring the food to your mouth (and not the other way round!).

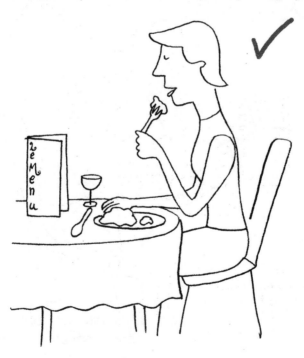

Of course, these ideas do not just apply to when we are eating out – this is not a book about etiquette! We need to be just as aware of how we eat when having a meal at home.

2. IN THE CAR

There is often an urgency about journeys; especially the busy commute to work or the frantic school-run. But jutting out your chin and leaning forward won't make the journey go any faster.

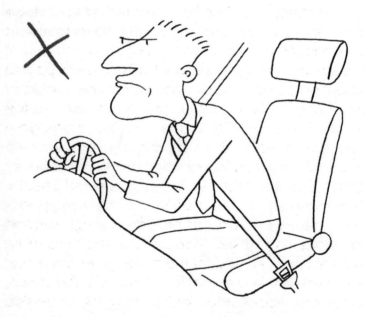

If we have habits of tension when we're eating in a restaurant, which is usually an enjoyable experience, how much more challenging might we find car journeys? A lot of frustrating factors might be making us feel negative, and our body use expresses this. You might be in your own car, but not one you would ideally choose; maybe it has badly designed seats, and perhaps the journey is tiresome and difficult, with traffic jams to contend with and children quarrelling in the back seat. But the journey has to be undertaken, so how do you keep feeling easy in your body with all these stressful factors?

If you are the driver, before you start off, think of that string attached to the crown of your head drawing you upwards. (You may have to adjust your mirror if you last made a journey at the end of a demanding day when you had *not* been paying attention to your body use: your spine wouldn't have been extended to its full length, and so the mirror would be tilted down to accommodate your shortened body.) Lengthening your neck will increase your peripheral vision, which is obviously going to be important to you as the driver (Chapter 8 Exercise 3). If the car seats are very poorly upholstered and do not provide enough support for your sitting bones, then invest in the hard foam wedges that are sold for the purpose. As the driver, your feet will need to make contact with the clutch, break and accelerator pedals. Allow the underside of your legs to lengthen as much as possible, using your feet on the pedals in an easy movement at your ankles and allowing your leg only the minimum tension required to keep the accelerator pedal pressed, tightening as little as possible at the knee and using the weight of your relaxed leg to keep the pressure steady. Let your hands rest easily on the steering wheel, with your arms relaxed and bent at the elbow.

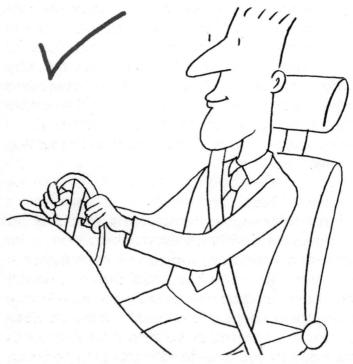

The passenger has a mechanically less complicated time, but of course being a passenger brings its own demands. Keep yourself unstressed by performing your own body check. You will have realised by now that the key areas are head and neck, shoulders and knees. So, like your driver, allow your neck to lengthen, but your hands can rest easily in your lap as you allow your shoulders to drop and widen and your legs to relax.

When the journey comes to an end, you will have to get out of the car, so how do you prepare to do this? Remembering to let your eyes lead your movement (as in the exercises in Chapter 8), turn your head first and then let your torso follow. Swivel your legs out of the open door and then let your feet contact the ground. Prepare to lift your body upwards by thinking of the buoyancy of your head and neck and taking the majority of the weight through your heels (as described in Chapter 13).

The same processes can be applied to journeys on public transport.

3. IN THE QUEUE

When standing in the bus or checkout queue, or working in occupations such as retail where a lot of standing is required, you can still draw from the same good standing habits detailed in Chapter 10 to make sure you are minimising tension in your body. Allow your spine to lengthen, be aware of the balance of your head on your neck, let your hands drop down by your sides to help your shoulders relax and make sure the weight of your body is evenly distributed between both feet. Most important of all, check that the majority of the weight of your standing body is referred down through your heels and NOT the balls of your feet.

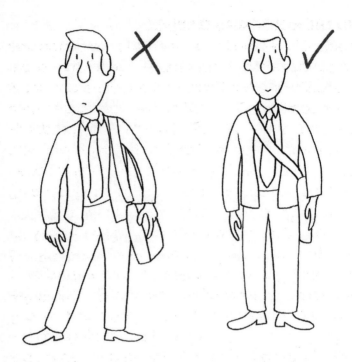

It is all too easy, when you are standing and waiting, to find yourself impatiently transferring too much weight forwards, or pushing a hip out to the side and transferring more weight onto one leg. If this happens your knees cannot help but be locked (and then your lower back tightens, followed by the rest of your spine).

Be cool, keep your weight central, and don't anticipate moving forward. When you do move and start to walk, remember (as in Chapter 10) that in poised walking your spine is carried along effortlessly, without lurching or thrusting forward.

4. IN THE HOUSE AND GARDEN

Check out your body use when you are performing routine domestic tasks. This is when the sheer mundanity and familiarity of the routine can show up our bad habits best! Often we want to get them over and done with quickly, and this produces unnecessary pressure. Just like the car driver who sticks out their chin to get to their destination faster, so we can become tense with the effort of doing the washing up. Just being aware of this possibility is a start. Observe yourself and notice how your neck, shoulders and legs feel. If you are working in a standing position where you are even *slightly* bent forward, remember the Post-it 'Use those knees' from Chapter 13. And, of course, in any bending and lifting, whether it is reaching into the fridge or pulling weeds up in the garden, remember the lessons learned in Chapter 13. Pay particular attention to how you are using your head and neck, shoulders and knees, and make sure you are sending your weight back down through your heels. This would especially apply to digging – a notorious cause of back pain. 'Put your back into it' is *such* a misleading phrase. The strength of a digging and lifting movement should come through your relaxed legs working as levers and lifting you, the spade and its contents up and down, with the weight dispersed predominantly through your heels.

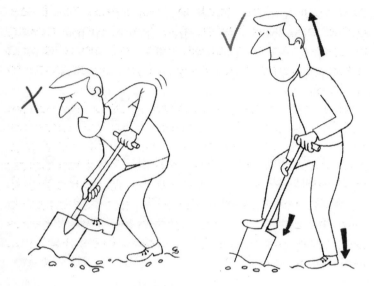

If boredom with the task in hand is a problem, combat it by reviewing the principle in Chapter 8 about staying focussed – you will benefit from giving attention to the job which has to be done.

5. GOING BY AIR

For many people, flying is the most stressful way to travel. It is nothing to do with being in the air, it's the process of getting on and off the plane which is so unpleasant. When you arrive at the airport, take time to be in the moment and stay focussed (as in Chapter 8). If you are carrying heavy bags, apply the lifting guidelines described in Chapter 13, which you should try to familiarise yourself with *before* you go on your journey. In the queue for the check-in desk, stand tall, relaxed, keeping your chest wide and your weight back in your heels. You'll feel better and look better. You never know; looking in command of yourself, with your relaxed and assertive demeanour, may get you an upgrade to business class!

When you finally reach your seat, unless you've got the upgrade, the chances are you may feel cramped and tense. Take a moment to relax and reorganise: think up, free the neck, widen across the chest and relax your knees (as far as the seat in front will allow). And whilst everyone else is fussing with the overhead bins, go through some of the breathing exercises in Chapter 14. There, don't you feel better already?

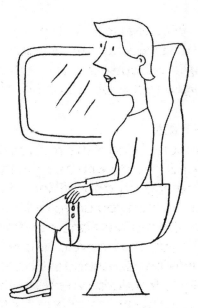

THE PRINCIPLE

The work you do on yourself is very much like a series of flight checks. You check out the key areas, which by now you will have recognised as your head and neck, shoulders and knees. In every situation you can bring your thoughts into your body to help you feel more physically at ease, and the easier you feel in your body, the easier you will feel in your mind.

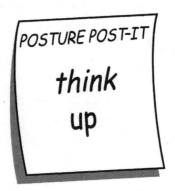

 REORGANISE YOUR LIFE

To get in control of your own body you have to put work into its re-education. Organise your time so that you are able to think through the exercises and principles in this book and inculcate them in your body and your life. So, even when you are in challenging and difficult situations you can meet them with a new attitude and approach. As you practise the exercises in this book and learn a new body vocabulary, you will find you have your own way of applying the principles to your own life. As you encounter new situations, think of all you have learned, but most especially think of your head, neck and back (i.e. your spine) working as one unit. In other words – think up!

Here's to a new, more poised and relaxed you.

CHAPTER 17

WHERE NEXT?

You never stop. As we said in the introduction, you keep working on yourself. You have learned damaging postural habits by repetition and repetition is the only way you will unlearn them. Repeat the exercises and continue to think about the way you move and perform everyday tasks. You never reach the end of the journey; there is always something new to learn, a new challenge to meet and a new situation to react to.

The exercises and ideas in *The Well-tuned Body* are predominantly derived from direct experience of the Alexander technique and the aim is to be both practical and useful. However, a book cannot be a substitute for experience. To experience the Alexander technique you need an accomplished teacher. The technique is a collaborative process and you will find the skills and insight of a good teacher absolutely invaluable.

You can find your nearest teacher of the Alexander technique by contacting STAT, the professional association:

The Society of Teachers of the Alexander Technique
(STAT)
Linton House,
39-51 Highgate Road,
London NW5 1RS
Tel: 0845 230 7828
Fax: 020 7482 5435
e-mail: office@stat.org.uk
website: www.stat.org.uk

The inspiration for much of this book has arisen from working with colleagues, friends and pupils. This, too, is an ongoing process and you can keep up with our latest ideas on our website at:
www.thebusybody.co.uk

APPENDIX 1

BODY MAP

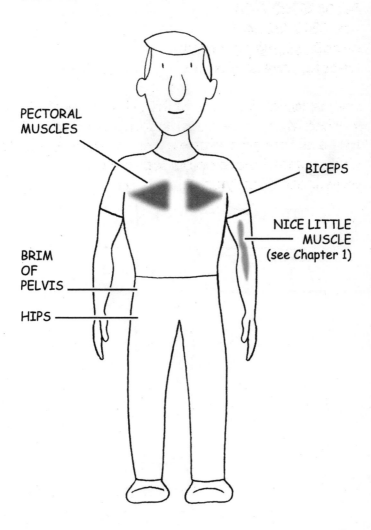

PECTORAL
MUSCLES

BICEPS

NICE LITTLE
MUSCLE
(see Chapter 1)

BRIM
OF
PELVIS

HIPS

THE WELL-TUNED BODY

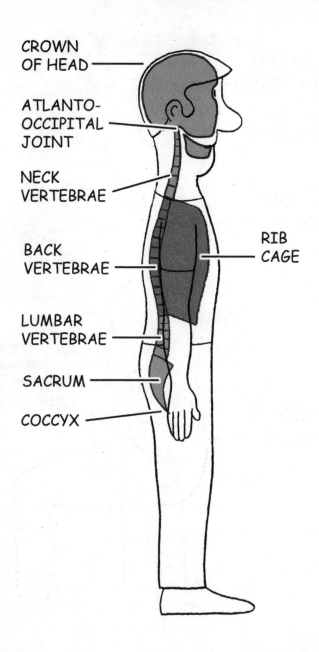

CROWN OF HEAD

ATLANTO-OCCIPITAL JOINT

NECK VERTEBRAE

BACK VERTEBRAE

LUMBAR VERTEBRAE

SACRUM

COCCYX

RIB CAGE

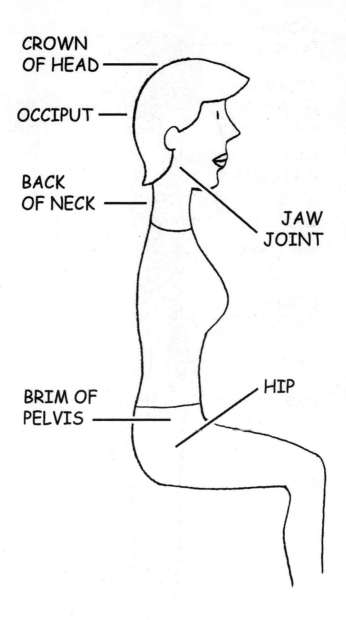

CROWN
OF HEAD

OCCIPUT

BACK
OF NECK

JAW
JOINT

BRIM OF
PELVIS

HIP

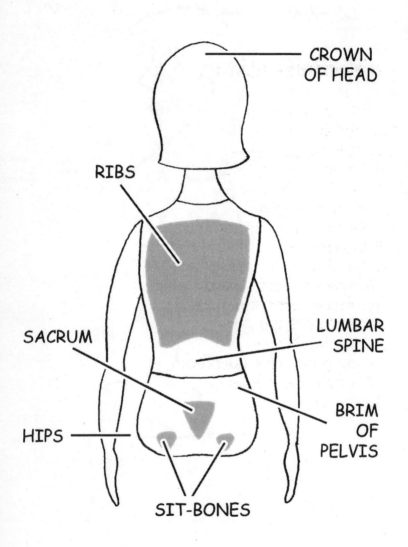

CROWN
OF HEAD

RIBS

SACRUM

LUMBAR
SPINE

HIPS

BRIM
OF
PELVIS

SIT-BONES

APPENDIX 2

THE POSTURE POST-ITS

1. Watch yourself
2. Stop and think
3. Think up
4. Lie down and recharge
5. Use those sit bones
6. Pivot at the hips
7. Relax and go further
8. Eyes lead
9. Simply does it
10. Move forward but stay back
11. Widen across the shoulders
12. Explore all the parts
13. Use those knees
14. Let go with the out breath
15. Stay in the moment
16. Think up

ACKNOWLEDGEMENTS

For his inspirational teaching, Don Burton, without whom this book would not have been written. Thanks to Wendy Bonington for her valuable feedback and to all other colleagues, pupils, students on courses and especially those at Cumbria Alexander Training who have, over the years, provided the catalyst for constantly developing the work. Thanks also go to our editor, Lucy York of Summersdale, for all her help in producing a well-tuned text. There are debts of other kinds to people in and out of organisations, including those who tried out and commented very usefully on our exercises as they were written: Edna Burnett, Ann Clark, Martin Condit, Gillian Cowburn, Martin and Jane Dix, the Hall family, Joyce Harris, Jane Howarth, Peter Leney, Judith Maddison, Kate Morpeth, Michael Mumford, Kathleen Purdy, Carolyn Stone and Helen Vaughan. To John Benson for his invaluable input to the revisions in this book, and to him and Pam Grant for putting up with us when we don't do as we say.

geoff thompson

stress
buster

how to stop stress
from killing you

Stress Buster
How to Stop Stress From Killing You

Geoff Thompson

£7.99

Paperback

ISBN 13: 978 1 84024 509 3

In our increasingly hectic society we are under constant pressure to get the best results, the top job, a better car or a bigger house. For many reasons, stress can become a major problem affecting our relationships and even our health. Stress can ruin lives, and most people don't know how to cope with it - or how they can use it as an energy force.

If you're always getting angry in the car, at home or at work, if you constantly feel out of balance, then this book is for you. It will help you identify the causes of stress in your life, and shows you how to deal with them in a practical way. With true-life examples, clear explanations and relevant advice, it is an indispensable aid to overcoming stress.

This book may save your life.

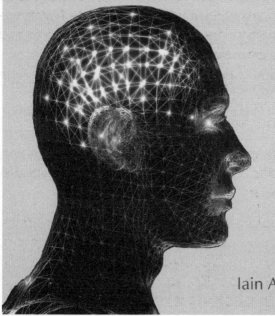

Mental
Strength

Condition your mind
achieve your goals

Iain Abernethy

Mental Strength
Condition your Mind to Achieve your Goals

Iain Abernethy

£9.99

Paperback

ISBN 13: 978 1 84024 324 3

Many people have dreams they would like to realise and things about their lives that they would like to change. However, relatively few people have the mental strength to break outside their comfort zone and to take the steps needed.

Fear, self-doubt, lack of confidence, or simply being overawed by the tasks ahead can stop you achieving your true potential.

There is nothing we cannot achieve and nothing we cannot become if we have the mental strength needed to reach our goals.

Mental Strength gives clear, encouraging guidance on how to develop a strong and powerful mind, grow your talents, become the person you want to be, and live the life you want to live. For the mentally strong, nothing is impossible!

www.summersdale.com